Research Report No 15

Teenage Mothers and Their Partners

A survey in England and Wales

Madeleine Simms and
Christopher Smith

Institute for Social Studies in Medical Care

LONDON: HER MAJESTY'S STATIONERY OFFICE

HQ
159.4
55

HMSO publications are available from:

HMSO Publications Centre
(Mail and telephone orders only)
PO Box 276, London SW8 5DT
Telephone orders (01) 622 3316
General enquiries (01) 211 5656

HMSO Bookshops
49 High Holborn, London, WC1V 6HB   (01) 211 5656 (Counter service only)
258 Broad Street, Birmingham, B1 2HE   (021) 643 3757
Southey House, 33 Wine Street, Bristol, BS1 2BQ   (0272) 24306/24307
9-21 Princess Street, Manchester, M60 8AS   (061) 834 7201
80 Chichester Street, Belfast, BT1 4JY   (0232) 234488
13a Castle Street, Edinburgh, EH2 3AR   (031) 225 6333

HMSO's Accredited Agents
(see Yellow Pages)

And through good booksellers

ISBN 0 11 320860 X

Contents

Preface

Teenage women can follow one of three paths. They can continue their education and training, if they have the opportunity and are sufficiently able and motivated, and aim at a career and status some time in the future; or they can enter the world of work as soon as they reach school leaving age, acquiring usually an office or semi-skilled manual job, with some money and some degree of immediate independence, provided a job is available; or they can have a baby. This too, will achieve for them adult status of a kind, whether or not they marry or cohabit with the baby's father.

This book is about this third group, who became mothers very young, before the age of 20. These three groupings are not, of course, wholly exclusive. Two-fifths of our sample of teenage mothers had managed to acquire at least one CSE before leaving school, and one-fifth had obtained at least one 'O' level. Rather more had worked at least briefly in clerical or semi-skilled jobs between leaving school and having a baby. But these were incidents on the path to motherhood. Education and work, so dominant in the lives of the majority of teenagers in this country, played little part in the lives of these teenagers whose principal role was that of mother.

This book is about the problems that face teenage mothers in the 15 months after the birth of their baby. It is not an encyclopedia about teenage mothers. It does not aim to provide all the available information about mothers in this age group. Nonetheless, in each chapter we try to outline the context into which to fit the problems we have uncovered. We have also tried, wherever possible, to make social policy suggestions relevant to the problems that have emerged in the course of this study. We hope the book will interest all those who come into frequent contact with teenage mothers and their families and who try to help them to sort out the difficulties they sometimes face in becoming mothers so young.

This book is also, to a lesser extent, about the partners of these women, the fathers of their babies, who were also mostly young. This is an elusive group about whom not very much is known: we thought it worth trying to find out as much as possible about them even though we were unable to interview as many as we would have wished. So this part of our investigation must be considered tentative and experimental.

We are grateful to the Department of Health and Social Security for supporting this study, and to Ann Cartwright and colleagues at the Institute for Social Studies in Medical Care who read and commented on the work in progress, particularly Rob Anderson, Claudia Martin, Ann Jacoby, Danny Kushlick and the Institute's Advisory Committee. We would also like to thank Anne Klepacz and her colleagues at the Office of Population Censuses and Surveys for undertaking the sampling and the interviews,

Heather Taylor for undertaking the onerous task of typing the text, and the young mothers and their partners who gave their time so generously. However, the views expressed in the course of this book are those of the authors alone.

Finally, we would like to acknowledge with thanks the editors of the following journals who have allowed us to reprint material that originally appeared in their columns:

Adoption and Fostering
British Journal of Sexual Medicine
Family Planning Today
Health Education Journal
Health Visitor
Journal of Obstetrics and Gynaecology
Marriage Guidance
Maternity Action
Midwife, Health Visitor and Community Nurse
Modern Medicine
Nursery World
Roof
Youth-in-Society

Thanks are likewise due to Lorna McKee and Margaret O'Brien, the editors of The Father Figure published by Tavistock Publications.

Madeleine Simms and Christopher Smith
London, 1985

1 Introduction

The purpose of the study

In this study we have looked at a random sample of teenage mothers in England and Wales to find out how they came to have their babies so young, how they fared with their babies in the first year-and-a-quarter after the birth, what the changing circumstances of their lives were during this period, and what they thought about their experiences in retrospect. We also carried out a similar, though more limited, survey among the fathers of the babies.

Our purpose in undertaking this study was to find out how the youngest group of parents in our community cope with the first stage of parenthood in the expectation that this information may ultimately have some bearing on social policy in relation to sex education, housing, the medical, social, family planning and other services affecting this age group.

Background to the study

Some facts and figures

In the decade between 1970 and 1980 some 83–104,000 teenage girls became pregnant each year in England and Wales. But, whereas in 1970 81,000 had babies and only 15,000 had abortions, by 1980 only 61,000 had babies while 36,000 had abortions. The fertility rate had fallen from 50 to 31 per 1,000 teenage women (OPCS, 1977 and 1982), while the abortion rate had doubled from nine to 18 per 1,000 (Bury, 1984). So why was a study of this kind thought to be necessary when teenage motherhood was no longer a growing phenomenon? Indeed, on 12 June 1984 the Office of Population Censuses and Surveys published a Monitor reporting that 'at ages 15 to 19 the fertility rate in 1983 was the lowest since 1955' (OPCS, 1984).

There are two kinds of answer to this question. One concerns the increased risks to both mother and child of early motherhood. The other relates to the effects of early parenthood on the future life chances of the young parents, and in particular of the young mothers.

Medical risks

Childbearing teenagers, particularly in the younger age groups, suffer more than mothers in their early twenties from a number of medical conditions including hypertension, toxaemia, anaemia (Russell, 1981; Zackler and Bradstreet, 1975) and pre-eclampsia (British Medical Journal, 1975) and are therefore more at risk of giving birth to vulnerable and 'small-for-dates' babies for every period of gestation.

The British Births 1970 survey (Chamberlain et al., 1975) refers to the 'well established pattern' of higher perinatal mortality in very young and relatively old mothers, and shows that in 1970 perinatal mortality per 1,000 births was nearly 29 for the under twenties compared with 18 for women in their early twenties. By 1980 there had been a great fall in overall perinatal mortality rates but the differences between the age groups were still present. The rate for mothers aged between 16 and 19 in England and Wales was 17 per 1,000 and for those in their early twenties 13 per 1,000. However, among the less than 1,300 births to girls aged under 16 years the perinatal death rate was 19 per 1,000. Stillbirths, neonatal deaths, post-neonatal deaths and infant deaths all follow much the same pattern of being somewhat higher for the teenage group than for the 20–24 age group (OPCS, 1982a).

In a recent study (Osbourne et al., 1981) it was suggested that improvements in obstetric practice over the past decade have had a positive effect on the outcome of teenage pregnancy. In the sample studied, anaemia was the only ante-natal complication that was significantly greater for teenagers than for those aged 20–24 years. However, being unmarried constituted an additional risk factor for this age group:

'Those who remained single showed significantly higher rates of premature labour and perinatal mortality when compared with the married women, and appear to constitute an at-risk group.'

Psycho-social risks

In addition to physical risks, there are also psycho-social risks to be taken into account. Rimmer (1981) observes that 'marriages in which a bride is in her teens are about twice as likely to end in divorce as marriages where the bride is in the age group 20–24, and four times as likely as those in which the bride is in the 25–29 age group'. Rutter (1979) says:

'Children whose birth was not wanted by their parents, who were born to teenage mothers, who were brought up in single parent households, and who grew up in very large families, are all subject to a substantially increased risk of psychosocial problems.'

He points out that the rate of depressive disorders increases sharply during adolescence, which may make pregnancy at this time additionally problematic. Moreover teenage pregnancy is associated with illegitimate births—in 1980 a third of all illegitimate births were to teenage women (OPCS, 1982)—and this in turn is associated with all kinds of deprivation (Committee on One Parent Families, 1974). Smith et al. (1973) and Baldwin and Oliver (1975) have noted that the parents of battered babies tend to be very young. In a recent study, (Taylor et al., 1983) it has been observed that the children of teenage mothers are much more likely to have accidents, both in the home and outdoors, than children of older mothers. These children had significantly more hospital admissions on this account. This remained true, even after allowance had been made for the inferior socio-economic circumstances in which these young mothers lived compared with older mothers. The authors conclude:

'. . . low maternal age is of itself a health hazard for children'.

In her comprehensive review of the literature Bury (1984) observes:

'Whatever the outcome, pregnancy in a teenager involves greater risks for the mother, and for the child if it is born, than pregnancy in an older woman. These risks are probably less than they were, due to better antenatal care and improved techniques of abortion. Many of the risks are associated with the adverse social circumstances of many of these teenagers but some risks, especially that of prematurity in the younger teenager, seem to be associated with age alone. Thus, although deferring pregnancy would lessen many of these adverse consequences, it would not eliminate them.'

Russell (1981) states his opinion that 'nothing about these pregnancies is to the advantage of the girls or their families' and goes on to say of the under-16s who become pregnant, that they do so:

'. . . before they have much idea of what life has to offer. And next to nothing is known of the youths who father these pregnancies; mostly they avoid any significant involvement in the problems raised by the pregnancy, leaving the girl and her family to sort things out as best they can.'

An editorial in the British Medical Journal (1975) also stressed the social problems and social dislocation of which teenage pregnancy was seen both as a symptom and a cause:

'The same sorry tale of broken homes, breakdown of family life, and poor education, as well as failure of education about contraceptives to reach those most in need of it.'

Effects on lifestyle and economic opportunities

In addition to the practical medical, social and psychiatric factors mentioned above, more fundamental objections to parenthood at this age are some-times made. These centre on the sudden curtailment of choice about lifestyles, jobs, partners and futures that early pregnancy brings with it. It is argued that the moment a teenager becomes a mother, her chances of advancement in worldly terms, and of widening her horizons in personal terms, come in most cases to an abrupt end (European Collaborative Committee for Child Health, 1983). Wealthy teenagers may, of course, evade these limitations with the aid of the services money can buy. Despite having a baby so young, their lifestyle would not be cramped, their housing would not be affected, they could obtain domestic and nursery help and continue their education, travel and cultural development. But such cases are few; the vast majority of teenagers who have babies come from the lower social classes (Kiernan, 1980; Wilson, 1980; European Collaborative Committee for Child Health, 1983) and do so, it is suggested, at the cost of a sudden and sharp restriction in the kinds of choices they can make about their own lives in the future.

It is sometimes argued that many working-class teenagers in our society have few choices or chances to begin with, so they may have little to lose. Thus, for them, teenage parenthood may not seem so negative as it might for a more fortunate middle-class girl whose alternatives, at any rate until recently, were a variety of training and educational possibilities followed by a variety of work or career opportunities. Such a girl may also reasonably look forward to saving some money and setting up an independent home before embarking on motherhood. If however, none or few of these alternatives face a woman with little education and few skills, as most teenage mothers have (Kiernan, 1980; European Collaborative Committee for Child Health, 1983) then perhaps her choice, if choice it is, of early motherhood, may have something to commend it? This dilemma is referred to by Bolton (1980) as the 'cruel problem' in that 'its most common victims are those persons within society who can least afford another attack upon their limited social, personal and economic resources'.

The young fathers

As pointed out by Russell (1981) little is known about the male partners of teenage mothers. Most, however, are also likely to be young. Data about the ages of the partners of teenage mothers are only available for legitimate births; in 1980 a fifth of all legitimate babies born to teenage women had teenage fathers and a further three-fifths had fathers aged 20–24 (OPCS, 1982b). Many are likely to be unemployed or in insecure low paid jobs. Evidence from America shows that men who father a child in their teens receive less formal education and show a lower occupational achievement than men who do not (Elster and Panzarine, 1981). It seems reasonable to suppose, therefore, that physical and social mobility and opportunities for training and advancement might also be curtailed for young fathers and that this might cause resentment and longer term problems.

American experience

In the United States, where one-fifth of all births occur in women aged under 19 years (Hollingsworth and Kreutner, 1980), teenage pregnancy is often referred to as an 'epidemic' (Alan Guttmacher Institute, 1976). Moreover, within the teenage group, the pattern of births is shifting towards the younger age groups. Studies there (Hollingsworth and Kreutner, 1980) confirm both the physical and psycho-social hazards noted in the English literature. In consequence, large sums of Federal money have been allocated to prenatal care for adolescents and to programmes for the prevention of unintended pregnancy. Adverse effects on the children of teenage mothers have also been noted, though these may be as much the effects of low economic status as of age:

> '. . . studies suggested that infants born to young mothers showed deficits in physical health, cognitive development, social/emotional development, and school achievement' (Klerman, 1980).

Public attitudes

There can be little doubt that an association between teenage parenthood and a variety of social ills exists in the public as well as in the professional mind. Hardly a week has passed since this research project started without startling headlines in the papers about 'The-Perils-of-Young-Love' (*Daily Express,* 27.9.79), 'Gymslip Mothers Shunned by the State' (*Daily Mail,* 20.4.79), 'The Young Love Charter' (*Evening Standard,* 11.9.79). 'Teeny-Mums' and 'Adolescents-in-Trouble' also figure frequently. There have been several television programmes on the subject and at least one national conference (Brook Education and Publications Unit, 1981). So whether or

4

not teenage pregnancy and parenthood really do constitute problems, they are certainly treated as such by the media and widely believed to be so by the public.

Study methods

This study, then, sought to investigate whether, in its early stages at any rate, teenage parenthood is as harmful a phenomenon as is widely believed, and if it is, what steps might be taken to mitigate it and to help other teenagers postpone or avoid it. To do this we needed a representative sample of mothers aged under 20 who had recently had a baby. The obvious source for such a sample was the Government's Register of Births. However, some parts of the birth certificate are confidential, including the age of the mother at the time of the baby's birth (though not, rather oddly, her marital status). So the sampling and interviewing had to be done by the staff of the Office of Population Censuses and Surveys, since they alone, under the terms of an Act of Parliament, The Population Statistics Act, are allowed to undertake confidential enquiries of this kind. Also the sample had to include a small number of ineligible, that is older, mothers to aid confidentiality. Thus in no individual case would the interviewer going on her rounds definitely know in advance that the mother was a teenager.

The sample was taken from births that occurred in 26 areas of England and Wales during July 1979. (The way the sample was selected is described in Appendix 1.) The interviewers from the Office of Population Censuses and Surveys first visited the mothers in their homes when the babies were two to four months old. Altogether, 86% (533) of the teenage mothers were successfully interviewed; 6% refused to be interviewed, the remaining 8% were always out or said it was inconvenient or had moved house or could not be traced. Those interviewed were asked if the interviewer could call on them again for further questioning in a year's time, and all but three mothers agreed to this. However, in the 15 instances where we found that a baby had died or been adopted before this interview, we did not call on the mothers a second time as we felt this would be too painful for them. Furthermore, many of the topics covered at this second stage were not applicable to these women.

In the event, we were able to re-interview 89% (456) of the women eligible for the follow-up stage, in the autumn of 1980. So, of the 623 teenage women who were selected for inclusion in this study, we managed to interview 533 (86%) the first time round, and 456 (73%) the second time round. This latter proportion rises to 77% if we exclude the women who were not eligible for the follow-up stage.

At both stages we used structured questionnaires, asking everybody the same questions. Most of the questions were factual, but some asked about their opinions and attitudes and could be answered at some length. The interviews lasted just over an hour on average and most of the teenage mothers were seen on their own.

Our sample was selected in such a way that it would, we hoped, be representative of teenage mothers in the country generally. Comparison with government information (OPCS, 1981 and 1981a) showed that we had a representative sample in relation to age and marital status. But more of

5

the babies in our sample had died within a year of birth (4% against 2% of babies born to teenage mothers nationally).[1] We also found that we had more British born women and more better off women among those we were able to interview compared with those we were unable to trace. (See Appendix 2.) So to this extent the conclusions drawn from our survey may be a little complacent. Had we been able to interview 100% of the women, we would probably have found out about the problems of more of the foreign born and poorer teenage mothers who live in England and Wales.

We also wanted to interview the fathers of the babies, if possible. So we asked the mothers if they minded. Most of the married women were quite happy about this and 93% gave us permission; but only 64% of the single women did so. Altogether we were given permission to interview 446 (84%) of the 533 fathers. Some of them, too, did not wish to be interviewed or were difficult to find. In the end we managed to interview 369 (83%) out of the 446. So of the 623 men who were eligible for inclusion in the study 59% were ultimately interviewed. Similar questionnaires were used as for the women though the interviews were rather shorter. Again, most of the men were interviewed alone.

Among the fathers we interviewed there was a lower proportion of teenage men, unmarried men, men in unskilled jobs[2] and men born in the West Indies than might have been expected had we managed to interview all 623 men. There was also a relatively low proportion of men who were not pleased about becoming fathers then and who were not involved in baby care. (The data are in Appendix 3.) So, once again, we may have a slightly rosy picture of the situation, but we have tried to allow for this in our conclusions.

Our sample of teenage mothers

So who are the teenage mothers in our study? Of the 533 women we interviewed a tenth were aged 16 or younger when they gave birth to their 'survey' baby and a fifth were aged 17. (Appendix 4 gives a description of the ten schoolgirl mothers in the sample.) The vast majority were aged 18 or 19. Two-thirds of the women were married by the time we interviewed them, though just over half of them had married since becoming pregnant with their 'survey' baby. As expected, the married women tended to be older than the single ones. This can be seen in Table 1.

The vast majority (92%) of the women had been born in Great Britain; 4% gave India, Pakistan or Bangladesh as their place of birth; and 4% came from other parts of the world. Ethnically, 91% were white Caucasians, 5% were Asians and 4% were West Indians. Two-thirds said they belonged to the Church of England or some other protestant denomination and around a tenth each said that they belonged to the Roman Catholic Church or that they belonged to some other religion or that they had no religion. Less than one-tenth said that religion was very important to them.

---

[1]Unless otherwise stated, attention has not been drawn to differences which might have occurred by chance five or more times in 100.

[2]Classification of social class is based upon the Registrar General's Classification of Occupations, 1970. The men have been classified on the basis of their own occupations, the women according to their father's present, main or last occupation.

Table 1 Age and marital status

Age at 'survey' baby's birth	Married before conceiving 'survey' baby	Married after conceiving 'survey' baby	Single	All women
	%	%	%	%
15 or younger	—	1	8	3
16	1	5	13	6
17	5	23	25	19
18	23	38	25	29
19	71	33	29	43
Average age	18.6	18.0	17.5	18.0
Number of women (=100%)*	161	195	174	533

*Small numbers for whom inadequate information was obtained have been omitted in this and in subsequent tables.

Family background

Studies have been carried out in Britain to establish whether those teenagers who become pregnant differ in terms of their childhood and adolescent experiences from those who do not (Kiernan, 1980; Wilson, 1980). These studies, as previously mentioned, show that teenage mothers tend to come disproportionately from working-class backgrounds. Whereas in 1979 only 59% of heads of household in Britain were classified as working-class (OPCS, 1981b), no less than 81% of those classified in our sample came from working-class families. So social class is one significant difference. Size of family of origin is another. The average size of the families of the women in our study was 4.4 children, which was more than twice the average number of children in families with dependent children in 1979/80 (OPCS, 1982c). Related to this is the high number of 'grandmothers' who themselves became mothers while they were still teenagers. In our study, nearly a third (29%) of the teenage mothers had mothers who had themselves started childbearing before the age of 20. In the nearest national comparison we can find (Dunnell, 1979), only 8% of women aged 35–49 had had a pregnancy by the time they were 20. Thus we were startled to discover that one in five of our 'grandmothers' were still in their thirties at the time of our first interview with their daughters, as were nearly a tenth of the 'grandfathers'. Also, one-third (35%) of the teenage mothers in our sample came from a broken home, where the parents' marriage had ended in separation, divorce or the death of a spouse. Interestingly, a higher proportion of the single teenage mothers than of the married ones came from a broken home (41% compared with 32%). By way of comparison, only 12% of families in Britain with dependent children were headed by a lone parent in 1979/80 (OPCS, 1982c).

Education and work

Educational achievement was another differentiating factor. Only 7% of our sample stayed on at school beyond the age of 16 years, compared with about 30% nationally. Whereas only 10% of all those leaving school do so without attaining any graded qualification whatsoever (CSO, 1982), more than half (52%) our sample fell into this category. This lack of educational achievement by teenage mothers is reflected in their occupations. Nearly half (46%) of those (80% of the total sample) who had had a full-time job were classified as having had a semi-skilled or unskilled occupation (waitresses, cleaners, laundry workers, canteen assistants etc.) whereas in Farrell's (1978) study, which was based on a nationally representative sample of 1,556 16–19 year olds, only 18% of working teenage girls were so classified (unpublished data).

Previous childbearing

An eighth (14%) of the women already had a child when they became pregnant with their 'survey' baby. Three women had already had two children. A tenth (11%) of the women had previously had miscarriages, induced abortions or stillbirths. So nearly a quarter (22%) of these teenage mothers had already experienced pregnancy before the birth of the baby that was the subject of our survey.

The 'survey' babies

Two hundred and seventy-nine of the teenage mothers in our sample had a boy, 249 had a girl, and five had twins. As expected, a slightly high proportion of the babies in our sample were of low birthweight; 9% weighed less than 2,500 grams compared with 6.7% of all live births in 1979 (Macfarlane and Mugford, 1984). Low birthweight is associated with premature labour and infant mortality. Not surprisingly, therefore, a relatively high proportion of the mothers in our sample described their baby as premature; 13% did compared with 8% in Cartwright's (1979) sample which was based on legitimate births to mothers of all ages. And, as previously mentioned, a relatively high proportion of the babies in our sample died within a year of birth; 4% did compared with 1% of all babies born in 1979. Four of the babies were adopted (see chapter 3) and three spent some time with foster parents during the first year-and-a-quarter of their lives.

Thus, teenage mothers tend to come from large, working-class families; their mothers have often started childbearing very young also. Many have experienced a broken home. Their educational achievement tends to be low and much of the work they engage in tends to be low status and poorly paid. Despite becoming mothers so young, a substantial minority have already been pregnant before. It seems, therefore, that teenage mothers in England and Wales tend to come from more deprived backgrounds than their contemporaries. How do they fare when faced with the responsibilities and problems associated with premature parenthood?

Overall impressions

Despite, or perhaps even because they tended to come from rather deprived backgrounds and to have led rather restricted lives, the majority of teenage mothers in our sample were delighted with their babies and their way of life and would not have it otherwise.

At the initial interview

Nearly all the women said they got on well with their parents; 96% said they got on well with their mother and 85% said they got on well with their father. Virtually all (95%) of those who were married described their marriages as happy—a view that was echoed by their husbands when questioned separately (see chapter 11).

Nine out of ten young mothers described their health as having been good since they got home from hospital with their 'survey' baby and four out of five said they did not go short of anything they needed. A similar proportion thought they were at least as well off as their contemporaries who generally had no children to support. Three-quarters thought their job prospects had not been affected by the pregnancy and about two-thirds thought their housing was suitable for their present needs (see chapter 7).

All but a handful of the women considered that their babies were easy to look after and less than a tenth (8%) wanted more help with their baby. The women derived great pleasure from having children and from watching them develop. Asked what they 'enjoyed most' about being a mother, they replied:

'Seeing him growing up and doing more things.'

'Seeing him smile . . . knowing he needs me . . . I can't really explain it.'

'Showing her off . . .'

'Just an inner feeling . . . It's looking at other women who haven't got any children. I've experiences the others haven't . . .'

One young mother replied ecstatically:

'Everything. I enjoy everything.'

Two-thirds of the teenage mothers thought things had worked out better than they had expected when they first found they were pregnant with their 'survey' baby. Nine out of ten thought things were going well for them and a similar proportion thought there was little they wanted to change about their current way of life. Only a fifth (21%) thought they would have any problems during the year following the initial interview and three-quarters were certain they wanted further children (see chapter 5).

One year later

Nearly nine out of ten women still said that, on balance, they were pleased they had had their 'survey' baby when they did. Though there had been some improvement in the women's housing situation between the two interviews (see chapter 7), one quarter (23%) said they were now worse off financially than the previous year. Additionally, the proportion who described their marriage as happy, the proportion who thought their 'survey' baby was easy to look after, the proportion who thought things had worked out better than they had expected when they found they were pregnant with their 'survey' baby, and the proportion who thought things were going

Table 2 Some differences in response at the two interviews

	At initial interview	At follow-up interview
Proportion who:		
described their marriage as happy	95%	86%
thought their baby was easy to look after	98%	91%
thought things had worked out better than expected	69%	60%
thought things were going very well	44%	30%
Number of women (= 100%)*	305	328

*As the table relates to more than one set of figures the minimum base number has been given.

very well for them, were all lower than in the previous year (see Table 2 for the data). Moreover, two-fifths (38%) of the women said they now went out less often in the evenings and at the week-ends than they had done a year earlier. Altogether, the picture was a little less rosy at the follow-up stage, than it had been at the initial one.

This book

The focus of the book is on social policy. We are therefore particularly concerned about the problems that teenage mothers experience in the course of bringing up their children. Consequently, most of this book is devoted to describing and analysing these problems: marital violence and breakdown, poor housing, depression and nerves, smoking, birth control failures and others. It is, however, important to bear in mind in reading about these problems, that the majority of teenage mothers in this study declared themselves well pleased with their lives and their babies, even though there was some decline in satisfaction with time.

2 Attitudes to becoming pregnant

There is a general impression that teenage pregnancies are unplanned and mostly unwanted. The abortion rate is higher for teenagers than for older women and in 1980 around a third of all teenage pregnancies ended in abortion (see chapter 1). Studies of mothers have shown that teenagers are more likely than older women to say their last pregnancy was unintended and to report an initially negative reaction to it (see, for example, Cartwright 1976 and 1978). But studies have also shown that for a not insignificant number of teenagers, pregnancy is a planned event (European Collaborative Committee for Child Health, 1983). In this chapter, we look at the attitudes of the teenage mothers in our sample to their 'survey' pregnancy. More specifically, we look at whether the women intended to become pregnant when they did, their use of birth control around the time they became pregnant, what their first reactions to the pregnancy were, and how their immediate family reacted to the pregnancy.

Intentions about 'survey' babies

Just over half (54%) the women described their 'survey' pregnancy as unintended. This proportion varied with marital status; it was 73% for single women, 63% for women who married after they became pregnant with their 'survey' baby and 24% for women who were married when they became pregnant with their 'survey' baby. Altogether 44% of the legitimate babies in our sample were described by their mothers as unintended which is somewhat lower than the 60% and 54% found by Cartwright (1976— unpublished data—and 1978) for comparable groups in her 1973 and 1975 surveys respectively. Although trends over time have to be interpreted with care, it does seem that in recent years the proportion of unintended babies born to married teenage women has been falling.

The proportion who described their pregnancy as unintended also varied with the age of the women, their social class, their ethnic background and the number of children they already had. It was relatively high for younger women (it fell from 80% for those aged under 17 to 45% for those aged 19), for working-class women (it increased from 44% for those classified as middle-class to 74% for those classified as social class V), for West Indian women (80% compared with 55% for white Caucasian women and 17% for Asian women) and for women having their first child (58% against 33% for those having their second or later child).

Use of birth control

Although over half the women said they did not intend to become pregnant, only a fifth of them reported using birth control around the time they

11

conceived. Of these women who were using birth control around the time they conceived, nearly a half had relied on the pill; nearly a third had relied on the sheath and most of the rest on withdrawal. Half of them ascribed their subsequent pregnancy to not taking or using their chosen method consistently or properly, while more than one-third said they thought the method itself was unreliable. They did not differ from the non-users in age or social class or the number of children they already had, but none of these women were Asian and a lower proportion of the married than of the single women were using birth control around that time (23% against 13%) presumably because the single women were the more anxious to avoid pregnancy.

The non-users

We asked the rest of the sample why they had not used birth control around the time they conceived. As expected, the reason many gave for this was that they had already decided to have a baby. Altogether 171 women (32% of the total sample) gave this as their reason while another 33 women (6%) said they did not mind having a baby even though they did not particularly want one, so that they were prepared to take risks with birth control. This rather casual attitude to the responsibilities of parenthood might be thought by many people to constitute a cause for concern. Occasionally the desire to have a baby had an ulterior motive:

'I wanted to have a baby because they would have to help me get a place if I had a family ... the Council are better if you've got a family ...'

Among those who were prepared to take a chance, the phrase 'we weren't bothered' was very common:

'Just didn't bother. Thought if we'd have a child—we'd have it ...'
'We were planning to get married. We weren't really bothered ...'
'I wasn't really bothered whether I had a baby or not, it didn't really bother me ...'

This, however, leaves two-fifths (42%) of the total sample not using any method of birth control, but not wanting a baby either. How did they account for this?

Pill problems

No less than 68 young women (13% of the total sample) said they had had problems with their previous method of birth control which had not yet been resolved when they found themselves pregnant. In nearly all cases these were problems with the pill, though the coil and the sheath were also mentioned a few times:

'I was taken off the pill. It was making me ill and I was due to have a coil fitted but it happened before that ...'
'I had cystitis and was asked to come off the pill and so I fell for the baby ...'
'Because I went off the pill as it was giving me depression and pains in the arms and chest. So I had to go off it and hadn't got round to anything else ...'
'I was told to come off the pill as it didn't suit me.'

12

'After using the Durex, he didn't like it. I went on the pill—I didn't like it. I got depressed on it—I couldn't be bothered to get up in the morning and lost several jobs because of this. I'm also a smoker and a drinker, so I gave up on the pill.'

Occasionally, the problems with the pill were anticipated rather than actual, and based on media reports and misreports:

'I didn't want to go on the pill because I read in the papers that this woman had jaundice and died, so I thought it might happen to me, so I didnt bother . . .'

In a few cases, the problems were with obtaining sheaths in time:

'. . . we couldn't always get them . . . I didn't go to the Family Planning Clinic and it was rather embarrassing buying them from shops . . .'

'that particular night we didn't have any . . . all the shops were shut.'

Dislike of birth control

Another 20 teenage mothers (4%) had thought about birth control but said they or their partner did not like using it:

'He couldn't get on with sheaths and I wasn't on the pill . . .'

'It's not the same . . . Durex you know . . .'

'We preferred it without using anything . . .'

'Well, I wouldn't go on the pill 'cos I was frightened, and he wouldn't use French letters as he didn't like it . . .'

'I didn't want a coil—to have something stuck inside me. With the pill, it makes some people fat and some people thin, so I didn't like it . . .'

Uncertain relationships 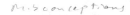 *misconceptions*

Another 18 women (3%) ascribed their failure to use birth control to the uncertainties of their relationship, or said it was the first time they had had sex so they did not know what to do:

'It wasn't really a regular relationship, it just happened once. I didn't think it was necessary . . .'

'I didn't know I could get pregnant . . . the first time won't harm . . . the first time won't do nothing, I thought . . .'

'. . . we had split up. Then we got back together for a short period . . .'

'I was on the pill first of all—then I split up with my boyfriend and came off the pill, and when I went back with him I didn't go on the pill again . . .'

Trusting the man sometimes proved a mistake:

'I think he did it for spite . . . he said he loved me and after that he never used anything. I kept saying what if I get pregnant but he said "so what" . . . he was willing to take the consequences and I thought if he doesn't mind, I don't . . .'

'Dunno—you think the chaps be safe . . . you trust them.'

Miscellaneous reasons

Thirty-three women (7%) gave a variety of replies that were hard to classify though some of these were very disturbing:

'I wanted to but he wouldn't let me. I wanted to take the pill but I knew if I did I'd get battered so thought better not than to keep having to go down to the doctors . . .'

'I did go to the family planning clinic but they sent me back to my own doctor who didn't want to know, and suggested I came back at a later date. When I did go back he found out that I was pregnant ...'

'My Dad wouldn't sign for me to go on the pill and I wouldn't use anything else ...'

There were worries about confidentiality. One woman said:

'I was going to go on the pill but I was a bit nervous my Dad was going to find out ...'

Two Rastafarians did not use birth control because they 'didn't believe in it'. One of these was 18 years of age, it was her second baby and her partner was in prison at the time of the initial interview. The other was 19 years and pregnant for the third time. Neither said they actually wanted a baby but were fatalistic about it.

Another woman remarked:

'It's silly really. I kept saying I would, but I never got up the courage to go to the doctors ...'

'I was scared to go and ask',

said yet another.

The don't knows

No less than 48 women (9%) said that using birth control had simply never occurred to them:

'it never entered our minds.'

'... never crossed my mind I could get pregnant.'

'I never thought about it ...'

In addition to these women, there were another group of 33 (6%) who replied 'don't know' in one form or another and whom, in reality, it is quite hard to distinguish from those to whom birth control had never even occurred.

Initial reactions

Clearly many of the women who had been having unprotected intercourse did not intend to become pregnant. However, not all of the women who described their pregnancy as unintended were displeased when they first suspected they might be pregnant. In fact, a quarter (23%) of them said they had been initially pleased about the pregnancy. The proportion for the women who described their pregnancy as intended was 83%.

Altogether half of the women said they had been initially pleased about the pregnancy:

'I thought it was great. I was over the moon.'

'I was happy. I wanted to go out and tell everybody I was pregnant.'

Two-fifths (39%) said they had mixed feelings:

'I thought it was quite good. I was a bit worried. Well, we weren't married and rather young but I was thrilled. I suppose I was a bit shocked. I didn't think it would happen to me.'

A tenth said they were upset or very upset:

'Shocked. I wasn't ready for that kind of thing you know. I went hysterical.'

And 1% made some other comment.

The proportion of women who initially had mixed feelings or were upset about their 'survey' pregnancy varied with marital status; it was higher for those who were single when they conceived than for those who were married at that time (63% against 20%). It was also relatively high for women aged under 18 (64% compared with 44% of other women) and for women having their first child (52% cf 32%) but it was relatively low for Asian women (28% cf 50%).

The parents' reactions

As might be expected, the women's parents were less likely to be pleased about the pregnancy than they themselves were. In fact, 43% reported that their mother was initially pleased about their 'survey' pregnancy. The proportion for fathers was 41%:

'She was pleased, she was all prepared to get the knitting needles out and start straight away.'

'Very pleased. He always said he couldn't wait for his first grandchild.'

A further 29% reported that their mother, and 24% that their father, initially had mixed feelings about the pregnancy:

'She weren't too bad but she was a bit worried 'cos I was too young and wouldn't be able to cope.'

But 26% reported that their mother was initially upset about the pregnancy and 30% that their father was:

'She could kill—she went mad. She was really upset 'cos I'm the only one and she wanted a proper Italian wedding with all the trimmings. She was hysterical. If she had a shot gun she would have blown my head off.'

'At first he wouldn't speak to me and wouldn't talk or have a fag with me and if he made tea I didn't get any. My Mum talked to him and he was OK but he was upset and thought I was stupid but it was only because he loved me that he cared.'

Two per cent made some other comment about their mother's reactions and 5% did so about their father's reactions.

Parents whose daughters were married were relatively likely to be reported as being pleased about becoming grandparents, as were middle-class parents, Asian parents, those whose daughters were in their late teens and those whose daughters were having their second or later child. The data are in Table 3.

Summing up

The women were asked a number of questions about their attitudes to their 'survey' pregnancy. Taking their responses to these questions together, showed that 35% of the women in our sample had a consistently 'positive' attitude to their pregnancy in so far as they had intended to become pregnant, had not used contraception around the time they became pregnant

Table 3   Some variations in parents' initial reactions to the pregnancy

	Mother pleased	Father pleased	Number of women (= 100%)*
Marital status:			
single	19%	15%	141
married after conceiving 'survey' baby	31%	30%	158
married before conceiving 'survey' baby	82%	81%	127
Social class of family of origin:			
middle class	55%	51%	78
III manual	41%	40%	220
IV	42%	32%	72
V	26%	26%	31
Ethnic background:			
white Caucasian	41%	38%	388
Asian	91%	95%	21
West Indian	(21%)	(29%)	17
Age:			
under 17	12%	7%	42
17	29%	19%	74
18	39%	42%	128
19	58%	55%	184
Parity:			
0	40%	37%	374
1 or higher	62%	65%	54
Total sample	43%	41%	428

* As these base numbers relate to more than one set of percentages, the minimum has been quoted.

and were pleased when they first realised that they might be pregnant. At the other end of the spectrum, just a few women (3%) had a consistently 'negative' attitude to their 'survey' pregnancy; these women had not intended to become pregnant, had used some method of birth control around the time they became pregnant and were upset when they first realised that they might be pregnant. This leaves the majority of women (62%) with either mixed feelings when they first realised that they might be pregnant or intentions which were inconsistent with their reactions to the pregnancy.

The proportion of intended and initially welcomed pregnancies in this study may, however, be an overestimate for the population studied. Furstenberg (1976) found that in general teenagers become more positive about their pregnancy as it proceeds. In this study, the teenage mothers were first interviewed when their babies were between two and four months old. Initial feelings of gloom may, therefore, have been dissipated by a process of accommodation to the pregnancy and the arrival of the baby. Furthermore, it is probable that a disproportionate number of the women we failed to interview had a consistently 'negative' attitude to their 'survey' pregnancy.

16

3 Unwanted babies: abortion and adoption

In the previous chapter we saw that a tenth of the women in our sample were initially upset about their 'survey' pregnancy while a further two-fifths had mixed feelings. Teenage women such as these who are not pleased about becoming pregnant have three options; they can reconcile themselves to the pregnancy and become a teenage mother; they can try to have their pregnancy terminated; or they can continue with the pregnancy and give the baby up for adoption. In this chapter, we look at the extent to which the women in our sample considered the last two of these options—abortion and adoption.

Abortion

Seventy (13%) of the teenage mothers in our sample said they had thought about having an abortion. At the time they became pregnant, around nine out of ten of these women were single, described their pregnancy as unintended and said they initially had mixed feelings or were upset. Nearly all (61) of these women had discussed the possibility of having an abortion with someone else. In the event, more than half these women did not pursue, or were deterred from pursuing an abortion after talking to a doctor, their parents, their partner or their friends.

Doctor: 'He said the hospital wouldn't do it so I'd have to pay. He just said they'd have no sympathy for me so I'd have to go privately.'

'The doctor said it could be too late to get rid of it. He said if I had an abortion it might come out alive and they'd have to keep it alive. I was 20 weeks.'

Mother: 'Mum was against it. To her it's murder. She doesn't like the idea at all. She promised to stand by me.'

Boyfriend: 'He didn't want me to have an abortion and suggested that we got married.'

Friend: 'Well about two years ago she had one. She just told me you don't feel very good for a few months afterwards. Mind you when I saw her she looked like a ghost after it.'

One woman reported that she approached the anti-abortion organisation Lifeline for help, possibly in ignorance of its views, and was informed that an abortion would cost '£95 plus VAT', which she could not afford. She continued with the pregnancy and the baby died soon after birth.

Other women who had thought about having an abortion decided not to pursue this option on moral or emotional grounds:

'I thought it was another little person that I had in myself and I would be destroying it.'

'I'd always think it was our fault. The baby didn't ask to be there, so why should you get rid of it.'

While some others said they eventually came to terms with being pregnant:

'After a while I thought I could cope like. I started to accept the fact like.'

'That depression thing only lasted a couple of weeks and when I'd got out of it I couldn't understand why I thought about it anyway.'

The women who sought an abortion

Twenty-four women (5%), however, said they had sought an abortion. One of these women confessed she never had the slightest intention of having an abortion and only applied for one in order to pacify her father who was outraged by her pregnancy.

The women who changed their minds

Eight women changed their minds and decided not to pursue the abortion mostly because they decided they wished to have a baby after all, or for reasons of inertia:

'The appointment was made for me to have it and I just didn't go ... My sister-in-law had an abortion and I saw what had happened to her. She was very, very depressed. She got to the stage that if she saw anyone else's baby she said it was hers; so I didn't want that to happen to me.'

Occasionally their boyfriends had a prevailing influence. One teenager had been pressured into applying for an abortion by the boyfriend who threatened not to go out with her again if she continued with the pregnancy. Another teenager withdrew from the abortion she wanted, at her boyfriend's insistence.

The women who attended 'too late'

Of the remaining 15 women (3% of the total sample), ten were informed by their doctors that they had come 'too late'. What stage of gestation their doctors regarded as 'too late' is not known with any certainty, though it is possible to make inferences from their replies to other questions. In response to the question 'When did you first see the doctor about your pregnancy—or about the possibility that you might be pregnant?' six women replied between five and nine weeks. One woman revealed that when she had first seen the doctor at eight weeks he said it would be too *early* to tell if she was pregnant. Yet when she went back for her next supply of contraceptive pills at 16 weeks he examined her and told her then it would be too *late* to have an abortion. Not only was this woman being seriously delayed, she was also evidently taking the pill while well on into her pregnancy. The remaining four women first saw their doctor about their pregnancy at between 13 and 18 weeks because they were 'embarrassed', 'scared', or had irregular periods and so did not realise they were pregnant.

One of the teenagers was so upset on being told she was 'too late' that she telephoned the hospital herself to try to obtain an appointment, but they apparently informed her that 'they did not agree with abortions'. She commented that she:

> '... didn't think it was right, didn't think it was fair. All my mind was upset ... I'd have one done now if I was pregnant again. I'd try my best to get one now that the baby hasn't even got a father.'

One girl was told she was too late for an NHS abortion and she would have to pay £200 to obtain one privately. She was given printed material explaining late abortions. This frightened her so much that she ran out of the office after ten minutes and left her social worker sitting there.

Another woman sensed that the gynaecologist to whom she had been referred was untruthful:

> 'He said I was too far gone and I knew he was lying. At three months I was too far gone and he couldn't perform the operation. I found out after that, that I was lied to. I wasn't three months pregnant. By her date of birth, I would have had her two months before if he had been telling the truth.'

Later, she reflected:

> 'I'm very pleased with her now but I don't think the doctor should have lied to me in the first place.'

The doctors who said 'no'

Five women reported that they were refused abortions by their general practitioners or gynaecologists without further explanations or on 'medical' grounds. For example:

> 'The doctor said I couldn't have one ... I didn't want the baby. He was making me bring the child into the world that I didn't really want at that time.'

> 'The doctor made the appointment. He explained everything in a letter to the hospital. They agreed there was no reason for me to have an abortion.'

> 'My doctor said I couldn't have one. He said I could go and see someone privately but he wouldn't want anything to do with it. But I didn't go after he'd talked to me. I got married. I might not be able to have any more (children) after an abortion ... I just took his advice.'

Thus, 13% of the women in our sample had considered having an abortion while 5% had made a serious and sustained attempt to obtain one. However, their requests for an abortion were turned down. Another way of confronting the issue of the unwanted baby is adoption.

Adoption

Seven per cent of our sample (37 women) said they had considered adoption at birth for their babies. Twenty of these women (54% compared with 10% of the rest of the sample) were so concerned not to have a baby to bring up at that time that they had also considered an abortion. Not surprisingly, therefore, the characteristics of the women who thought about adoption were similar to those of the women who thought about abortion. These 37 women who considered adoption were more likely to be single than the rest of the sample (76% compared with 29%) and were more likely to say their pregnancy had been unintended (81% cf 52%) and to have been initially upset about the pregnancy (30% cf 9%).

In the event, 26 of these women had pursued the matter to the extent of discussing this possibility with other people who included social workers, health visitors, welfare officers, parents, the fathers of the babies, and their doctors. Several had talked to more than one of these or to other people known to them. Husbands, boyfriends, and relatives were in general unenthusiastic about adoption, though one relative, an aunt, offered to adopt the baby herself and one mother tried to persuade her daughter to allow an infertile friend of hers to adopt the baby.

'He was against adoption because he didn't want me walking around for nine months pregnant, having it, seeing it, and then giving it away.'

Husband

'He didn't like it. He said we would get a house. He said it was ours and the council would have to give us a house.'

Boyfriend

(What she said was) 'Unrepeatable! She was dead against it.'

Sister

The professionals, on the other hand, generally left the mother to decide for herself, having offered her social work support and explained the legal procedures to her.

'She didn't say a lot. She let me do the talking. Really she said whatever I decided, she'd go along with me all the way.'

Social worker

One GP, however, was far from neutral. A 17 year-old mother reported:

'He was pleased, but when I said I had changed my mind he seemed to change from being very pleased to not ... He kept on so, that I changed my doctor.'

However, most of the women who thought about adoption eventually decided against this step. In most cases this was just a gut feeling that it was their child and could not be handed over to someone else:

'Once you hold them, you feel they are yours.'

'I just disagree with adoption. I don't believe a woman should have to go through such pain and then have to let her baby go.'

'I didn't want to go through all that just to give it away.'

One woman said she would feel guilty whenever the child's birthday came round. Another remarked that she needed the child for company. Another, whose second baby this was, observed:

'I thought, if I can manage one, I can manage another.'

Another said now she knew the baby, she was glad she had not had him adopted, but she reflected:

'I suppose I wouldn't have known what he was like if I'd had him adopted ... but now I'm glad I didn't.'

Another woman remarked:

'I think he deserved to know his own mother seeing he'd never know his father ...'

The women who favoured adoption

Altogether eight women decided to have their baby adopted at birth. For six of these women, however, the maternal instinct proved too strong and they changed their minds, some immediately and others after time for reflection had elapsed:

'I was given time to see if I could let him go, but I couldn't. I got him back. I just kept getting upset and depressed so I took him back ... I think I was mad ...'

'I left the baby at the hospital and I signed the papers and came home without her ... After three days I went back and collected her. I couldn't leave her. I wanted to bring her up myself. I went through the pain of having her.'

'Social worker came down and explained about it ... then she said it was up to me what I did. When he was born we decided to keep him ... I'm glad I never let him go.'

'Soon as she was born they just took her away. I never even saw her. They should have sent the forms in six weeks. I never got them. I rang up and said I'd changed my mind and wanted her back.'

'I went to the Adoption Centre twice and then, two or three weeks before I was going to have the baby I decided I wanted to keep it ... I'm glad.'

'I didn't want to see the baby but a student delivered it and he didn't know it was to be fostered. The next day it was beside the bed. I was upset about it. If I hadn't seen him I could have said—yes, adopt it.'

Two adoptions at birth

Two women had their babies adopted at birth. Both were unmarried and 18 years old when the baby was born. Both had been deserted by the baby's father as soon as he heard about the pregnancy.

One young mother lived alone with her parents in a small terrace house with only an outside lavatory. She worked full time in a textile factory, which she enjoyed, but the pay was low and she found money a problem. She said she had never intended to become pregnant when she did, was very upset when she first thought she might be pregnant, and had considered adoption from that moment on. She had also, briefly, thought about abortion and discussed this with a friend who had informed her that it would 'cost a lot', so she had dropped the idea. Asked why she decided to have the baby adopted, she replied:

'When I told my boyfriend, that was it, we were finished; and then I met someone else and he stuck by me and then I thought the baby would have a better chance with better clothes and everything, being adopted. It would have caused problems if I'd kept the baby. It would have been hard for (my) new boyfriend. He didn't want me to keep the baby although we told people I was pregnant by him.'

She now thought, looking back, that things had really worked out better than expected:

'I didn't think I would have the baby adopted. I thought my mum would force me to keep it and I didn't think they or my boyfriend would stick by me, and they have. I'm happier with my new boyfriend.'

She was hoping to become engaged next year and said that her advice to others in her situation would be:

'to have the baby and then make the decision about keeping it or having it adopted.'

She looked forward to having three children of her own, starting in two or three years' time:

'When I'm married, with a house—however long that takes.'

The other young mother lived in a semi-detached council house with her divorced mother and siblings. She worked in a shop and did additional evening work to earn extra money. When she first suspected she might be pregnant she thought:

'. . . if I didn't think about it, it would go away. Then I thought about abortion. But then I decided to go through with it and put it out for adoption, because with only my mother at home there would be no male figure for him.'

She said she decided to have the baby adopted because:

'There was no way the father would marry me. My mother was by herself . . . and it wasn't practical to have the baby. It would change my life too much . . . I wanted to give the baby the best possible start.'

Another factor, perhaps, was that her mother had once found herself in the same situation and married the man and it didn't work out:

'She didn't want me to make the same mistake.'

She was very pleased in retrospect that she had settled for adoption:

'If it had been secretive I would have always wondered about it, but everything was so open, I was even able to choose the parents, and my social worker was marvellous.'

She hoped to have four children in the future:

'I am getting married in two years time and I would like a baby straight away. It could be that I feel this having just had one adopted, but that's what I think at the moment.'

Two later adoptions

One year later when we called on the young mothers again, we found that two more of them had had their babies adopted.

One was a 17 year-old single woman, one of five children of an Irish Catholic mother who had died when she was only 12. This was her second child. At the time of our first visit, the young mother was living in a mother-and-baby home which housed 14 mothers and babies. Her aunt had advised adoption of the second child. She kept changing her mind about this, eventually agreed, but retrieved the baby after two months because she missed it.

When we revisited her one year later, it transpired that the baby had finally been adopted when it was about three months old:

'I couldn't cope with him—just too much with the two of them, being on my own.'

She had moved house twice during the year, and was now installed with one of her brothers and his family, with a new boyfriend and her first baby. She thought things were going well now and she hoped to have a third baby within a year, 'to take my mind off A—'.

The second mother was 18 and also single. Her aunt had offered to adopt the baby. She lived with her mother and sister in a council house. She had become pregnant unintentionally while drunk. Her boyfriend was a 15 year-old schoolboy. She wanted an abortion until she saw a television film on the subject:

'It put me off completely.'

Eventually, at five months, she did allow the baby to be adopted by the aunt:

'For what I got on the Social I couldn't keep up with him.'

Afterwards she felt 'awful' and often cried all night. So she became pregnant again almost at once, but had a miscarriage and felt even worse. She smokes quite heavily, ten to 20 cigarettes a day, and would like to have another baby within a year. She had had three pregnancies to date, one baby and two miscarriages.

Discussion

In 1979, when this study was carried out, the abortion rate was 17 per 1,000 teenage women (OPCS, 1981c). Our study suggests that this rate would have been higher if all the teenagers who had wanted to have an abortion had been able to obtain one. Some 3% of the women in our sample had actively sought an abortion but were either turned down by their doctors, generally without explanation, or were informed that they had applied for abortion 'too late', although six of the ten women in this last group had visited their doctor before they were ten weeks pregnant. This seems a cause for concern. Most of the women were unmarried, and five were only 16 or 17 years of age when they eventually had their babies.

Unlike abortions, the number of adoptions in Great Britain declined during the 1970's (CSO, 1982). This relative unpopularity of adoption in the late 1970's is reflected in our data; fewer women in our sample considered adoption than considered abortion. Altogether adoption was considered by 7% of the women in the sample, nearly three-quarters of whom discussed this possibility with others. In the event eight women decided to have their baby adopted at birth but six of these women changed their minds. The women who did have their baby adopted at birth seemed satisfied with their decision.

The two young mothers whose babies had been adopted at three and five months respectively were, however, both determined to have a baby again very soon to make up for their loss. This might suggest that these later adoptions were ill-advised and the mothers inadequately counselled. In one case the adoption occurred within the family, and it may have done so in the second case also. It seems that no social worker was involved at this later stage and that the adoptions were privately arranged. One wonders what the relationship between the teenage mother, the baby and the adoptive mother will be later on, since they will probably continue to be in touch with each other.

In addition to the four women we interviewed who had their baby adopted, there were nine women among the non-responders to our survey who also had their baby adopted (see Appendix 2). In these instances the girl or her family felt it would be too upsetting to bring up the subject again. It may be that these women, like the two women who had a late adoption, were finding it difficult to adjust to the situation. This might suggest that teenagers who give up their baby for adoption need more counselling and support than is presently realised.

4 The health and social services— ante- and post-natal care

ANTE-NATAL CARE

Teenage mothers are looked upon as a high risk group (see chapter 1) for whom contact with the health services early in pregnancy and beyond is usually considered desirable. Yet studies have shown that teenage mothers' use of ante-natal care services differs from that of older mothers in a number of respects. Unpublished data from Cartwright's (1979) study show that teenagers are more likely than older women to delay their first visit to a doctor until they are 12 or more weeks' pregnant; and O'Brien and Smith (1981) found that teenagers are relatively likely to attend for their first ante-natal visit after the 20th week of pregnancy and to miss visits once they had embarked on this care. We therefore asked the teenage mothers in our sample about the ante-natal care they had received and the data we collected are presented in the first part of this chapter.

First consultation with doctors

Two-fifths (42%) of the teenage mothers in our sample first consulted a doctor about their pregnancy within two months of conceiving; a further third (31%) consulted a doctor for the first time during the third month of their pregnancy while a quarter (27%) were three or more months' pregnant before they consulted a doctor. When we asked this last group of women why they had delayed their first visit to their doctor, the answer we received from nearly half (45%) was that they had not deliberately delayed their first visit—they had not realised they were pregnant:

'I didn't know I was pregnant. I went to the doctor's because of my headaches and he said I was pregnant. I didn't believe him even though he had done a test. I bought a test myself for three pounds and did that as well.'

'I didn't really take much notice because it had just turned Christmas and my husband was putting on weight and I was putting on weight but I wasn't getting very fat so I didn't bother. There's always stages in your life when you miss periods.'

Sixteen per cent mentioned fear and/or embarrassment about consulting a doctor:

'I suppose I put it off as long as I could. I didn't really want to see him. I don't like doctors. I was frightened of what would happen blood tests and things.'

'Just scared to go to a doctor because my doctor might have started going on at me. Telling me that I was stupid and should have done something about it.'

'Because I needed courage. Just to go in and say "Doctor I think I'm pregnant"— with not being married.'

Fourteen per cent suspected they were pregnant but hoped that they were not, and did not want their suspicions confirmed:

25

'I was trying to put it off and pretend it wasn't there.'

'I didn't want to. I didn't want it confirmed.'

Fourteen per cent could not bring themselves to tell their parents about the pregnancy so didn't feel able to consult a doctor:

'I think it was because I hadn't told my Mum and I didn't want to go behind Mum's back until she knew.'

'I don't know. I just never went. It all boiled down to the fact that I was frightened to tell my Dad. The doctor wouldn't tell my Dad but someone would know.'

Some of these women thought that the doctor would tell their parents:

'I thought he was friendly with my Mum and I thought he might tell her so I made sure first.'

'I didn't want to. I thought it might get back to Mum—the doctor might tell her.'

Thirteen per cent didn't perceive the need to go any earlier:

'I was alright, I didn't have any sickness but I wanted some iron tablets so I went then.'

'I just never bothered—I never bothered with none of them. I was always alright. I didn't see the point of going.'

Four per cent did not want to be talked into an abortion:

'Because I wasn't 16. I was scared because I was only 15 in case he tried to take it away from me.'

'So that there was no possibility of me having an abortion. The doctor might have persuaded me not to have had it. Where I was living—with my Mum—we were overcrowded. Only two bedrooms and the house had been condemned for two years. We had rats.'

'I wanted to have him and I didn't know if Mum would have made me do something . . . I thought she'd make me have an abortion.'

Eight per cent of the women gave some other or no reason for not seeing a doctor when less than 12 weeks pregnant. A few women gave more than one reason.

It may seem strange that such a large proportion of teenage girls appeared not to realise they might be pregnant, for more than three months. However, taking this group together with those who did suspect pregnancy but did not want this suspicion confirmed, and those who were afraid to break the news to their parents, suggests that many of these late attenders were, in fact, reluctant mothers. Further analysis tends to confirm this view. As can be seen from Table 4, women who described their pregnancy as unintended and those who said they were upset when they first realised they might be pregnant were relatively likely to have consulted a doctor for the first time late in pregnancy. Thus the real motivation behind late first attendance to confirm a pregnancy may often be reluctance to face up to the fact of pregnancy for all kinds of personal, social and economic reasons. A reluctance to become a teenage mother may therefore result not only in a relatively high rate of teenage abortion but also in delayed ante-natal care for those who do in the event continue with a pregnancy. Doubt about medical confidentiality is another factor in causing delay. Teenagers do, it

Table 4 Late comers for ante-natal care

	First consulted a doctor when 12 or more weeks pregnant	First attended ante-natal care when 20 or more weeks pregnant	Number of women (=100%)*
'Survey' pregnancy described as:			
intended	19%	14%	234
unintended	34%	22%	282
Initial reactions to 'survey' pregnancy:			
pleased	20%	15% ⎫	265
mixed feelings	31%	20% ⎬†	207
upset	42%	23% ⎭	53
Had thought about having 'survey' baby adopted:			
yes	34% ⎫†	38%	34
no	26% ⎭	17%	489
Age:			
under 17	49%	38%	48
17	32%	20%	98
18	27%	15%	154
19	20%	15%	227
Marital status:			
single	38%	26%	170
married after conceiving 'survey' baby	28%	16%	195
married before conceiving 'survey' baby	12%	11%	158
Social class:			
middle-class	21% ⎫†	11%	90
working-class	28% ⎭	19%	371
Ethnic Background:			
white Caucasian	27% ⎫	19%	479
Asian	16% ⎬†	4%	25
West Indian	25% ⎭	25%	20
Total sample	27%	18%	526

* As these base numbers relate to more than one set of percentages, the minimum has been quoted.
† These differences did not reach the level of statistical significance.

appears, still need to be reassured that their doctors will not reveal confidential information to their parents.

Late comers for ante-natal care

Just over a quarter (28%) of the women first had ante-natal care when they were less than three months' pregnant and around a half had their first ante-natal visit in either their third (35%) or fourth (18%) month of pregnancy. But nearly a fifth (18%) of the women received no ante-natal care until they were five or more months' pregnant and four women (1%) received no ante-natal care at all. All these four women were single. One, aged 14, could give no reason for not having had ante-natal care. Another was too busy caring for a sick mother until she was half way through her pregnancy:

'I thought it was too late then.'

Another teenager, who was pregnant with her third child, remarked that she had not attended:

'Cos I know how to do it from before.'

The fourth teenager did not realise she was pregnant:

'When I took my little girl to him (her doctor) he asked why I was putting on weight and I said I thought it was the pill and he did too, I think.'

The baby was born prematurely and died.

One-third of the women in our sample had a gap of at least eight weeks between first seeing their doctor to confirm the pregnancy and their first ante-natal visit. One woman who did not go to ante-natal care until she was over five months' pregnant said:

'You have to wait for an appointment. You go to your doctor and he sends off for you to get an appointment. I was waiting to go, that's all. You can't go till you've got an appointment.'

And another late attender said:

'They didn't send for me until I was seven months.'

However, those who came late for ante-natal care were also in most cases (66%) those whose first consultation with their doctor had taken place late. So these two overlapping groups had very similar characteristics. The late comers for ante-natal care were among the more reluctant mothers who were more likely than the rest of the sample to describe their pregnancy as unintended and to have considered adoption. The figures are in Table 4 which also shows that late attendance was greater for younger than for older women, for single than for married women, for working- than for middle-class women and for white Caucasians and West Indians than for Asians.

Apart from delays in getting the pregnancy confirmed and in being given the first appointment, embarrassment, moving house and work were given as reasons for late attendance at ante-natal care. In addition some women could see no point in early attendance for the healthy:

'No need. They only mess you about and examine you. If you're bad that's a different thing. Then you need to go.'

Missed visits

Altogether 80% of the women had some ante-natal care from a hospital and 67% from a GP; 48% had some care from both. Fourteen per cent of the women said they had missed an ante-natal visit, mostly (70%) just one or two visits. However, by the time of the interview they may have forgotten some of the visits they missed or been unwilling to admit to this.

One-third of the women who reported missing ante-natal visits said this was due to ill-health, and one-fifth mentioned problems of access:

'Our car broke down and when I got heavily pregnant I was unable to cycle to the clinic. Finally an ambulance took me to the local hospital for my check-ups.' (Missed four visits)

'It's an awkward place to get to. Not only that, I didn't have any money to get there. It's 80p odd return on the bus.' (Missed five visits)

28

One-fifth said they simply forgot some of their appointments. Some (12%) said they were too busy; some (8%) had difficulties making arrangements for their other children; some (7%) didn't see the necessity of going every time:

'I think I'd know myself if anything was wrong.'

And some (8%) disliked going for ante-natal care.

Attitudes to care

Women who missed ante-natal visits were less likely than those who did not, to say they were satisfied with their ante-natal care (62% compared with 81%). Altogether, 79% of the women declared themselves satisfied with the ante-natal care they were given:

'It was very good. They told you an awful lot and if you had any problems they'd explain it all to you. Very friendly.'

Fourteen per cent had mixed feelings while 7% were dissatisfied with their ante-natal care. Waiting time was an issue here—it was mentioned by two-fifths of the women who were dissatisfied with their care:

'It was silly. You had to wait from nine to one just to have a blood test and for them to take your blood pressure.'

'Always had to wait hours—never any different. I don't know why they made appointments, they never keep them. Dozens of us would be sitting there waiting for doctors to turn up.'

Another criticism, again mentioned by two-fifths of the women who were dissatisfied with their care, was that information was not readily given:

'Maybe I got the wrong idea from what you see on TV but I thought they would tell you things without being asked but they never did. I felt like a machine being weighed and tested.'

'They didn't tell you much, it's as if you weren't supposed to know anything.'

The third most frequently voiced complaint by these women who were dissatisfied with their ante-natal care was that the clinic was overcrowded. This was mentioned by a fifth of them:

'I was alright at the doctors but I hated going to the hospital. When you were there it was packed, you couldn't get a seat, you were all hot and bothered and didn't know where you were ... You didn't dare go to the toilet in case you missed your turn.'

Other criticisms made by the women who were dissatisfied with their ante-natal care included seeing a different doctor or midwife at each visit, and receiving conflicting advice.

Comment on ante-natal care

More than one-quarter of the teenage mothers in our sample consulted their doctor for the first time when they were more than three months pregnant, and one-fifth did not arrive for their first ante-natal visit until they were more than five months pregnant. As noted, these two groups overlapped to a great extent. Once a young pregnant women delays her entry into medical care, due in most cases it seems to ambivalence about the pregnancy or a reluctance to face motherhood, then the subsequent delays in the system will ensure that in many cases she also comes late to ante-natal and hospital care. One-third of the sample had at least a two month gap between seeing their family doctor to confirm the pregnancy and their first official ante-natal visit. There were complaints about long waits for attention, sometimes resulting in the women returning home without being seen by a doctor, or in subsequent missed ante-natal visits. There is clearly a failure in management here. It would surely be more satisfactory from everyone's point of view if those patients who were not judged to be in a very high risk category, were required to attend for ante-natal care less frequently, but were seen more promptly and offered more time, attention and discussion when they did come. Hall et al. (1980) in a survey in Aberdeen have arrived at a similar conclusion though for somewhat different reasons:

> 'The productivity of routine ante-natal care in respect of prediction and detection of obstetric problems is extremely low, and it is suggested that the number of visits for this purpose could be considerably reduced for women without special problems.'

At the moment, about one-fifth of all teenage mothers look back on their experience of ante-natal care without very much satisfaction. Perhaps one reason for this is that some young women are being urged to attend more often than is really necessary, but are not treated with the attention and consideration they expect when they do attend. Given the difficulties some young women have to overcome in order to be able to attend regularly, this seems unfortunate, and it may be that the proposal put forward by Hall et al. (1980) that 'ante-natal clinic visits should only take place if an objective can be specified with a reasonable expectation of being met' is one that requires to be taken seriously with this age group as with older pregnant women.

POST-NATAL CARE

In the second part of the chapter, the contacts the teenage mothers had with the health and social services in the first few months after giving birth are examined. Discussion is centred on their contacts with GPs, health visitors, social workers and baby clinics.

General practitioners

Eighty-seven per cent (466) of the teenage mothers had seen their GP between the time they got home with their baby and the initial interview. Nearly all these women (88%) had positive things to say about their GP, three-fifths describing him or her as very helpful. Of the women who had not seen their GP, only three said they would have liked to have seen him or her. Two of these three women wanted advice about birth control.

This section is about the small proportion of women (12%) who reported that they did not for one reason or another find their GPs helpful. The age distribution of this 12% (55 women) was similar to that of the rest of the sample as was the proportion who were married.

30

Lack of interest

The most common complaint, voiced by 22 women in this small group, was of 'lack of interest' shown sometimes by failure to examine, or by resort to routine medication:

'He just said "Where's the baby", and I told him he was in the cemetery. He just wasn't taking any interest . . .' (Mother whose baby died.)

'The only thing he could do was give drops . . .'

'He never looked at him (the baby)—just gave him a prescription . . .'

'When I went to see him for my post-natal he didn't check me so I got worried . . . he was on the 'phone all the time I was there. By the time he finished he'd forgotten all about me . . . I'm changing doctors.'

'The doctor didn't look at me and bustled me out with a prescription . . .'

'He just gave me some tranquillisers but he wouldn't write to them (Housing Association, as advised by health visitor) . . . he just wasn't interested . . .'

Problems of communication

It is sometimes difficult to disentangle lack of interest from failures in communication. Eighteen mothers complained that their family doctors seemed to go about their work in virtual silence, though six of them conceded that this could be due to sheer lack of time on the part of the doctors rushing from one patient to the next:

'He just doesn't say very much. He just goes in and out and that's it . . .'

'He doesn't seem very sociable. He was in such a hurry—straight in and out . . .'

'I like a doctor to talk to you but he wouldn't . . .'

'Hopeless—he didn't explain anything.'

One young mother summed up her feelings on this issue by remarking:

'If you've got any troubles you talk to your family, not doctors these days. Well, doctors used to be friends, but now they don't have time to be . . .'

Problems of treatment

Seven patients complained of the medical treatment they received. One of these reported that the baby clinic took over the case when the baby was in continuous pain, and helped solve the problem. Another said that the health visitor saved the day by her advice. One young mother said she had an extremely elderly GP who she thought no longer knew what he was doing. One woman, having been told by her doctor that she did not have an abscess, reported that she went to the hospital where they found it was an abscess and treated it properly, as she believed, for the first time:

'So I'm not very fond of that doctor!'

Another young woman ended up in hospital for treatment after her mother intervened, because the GP seemed to them incapable of listening to the problems or understanding what was the matter. The young mother was now going to transfer to another doctor. One young mother had had tablets prescribed for both stomach trouble and depression and remarked:

'The same doctor prescribed both so he should have known better. He should have known the two tablets didn't agree, seeing as he gave me both.'

In one case medical inadequacy was believed to have been compounded by clerical incompetence:

'When I went back it (abscess) hadn't cleared up. That was a week later and I was in agony, and there weren't any notes. There wasn't any record with my notes of what he'd given me. They were tablets to take every two hours and they asked me what they were, but I didn't know ...'

Other problems

Three doctors were seen as being actively unpleasant. One had a row with a young mother because she eventually decided to give up breastfeeding and go back to work. He told her what he thought about that in no uncertain terms, which went down rather badly as she alleged he had failed to visit her during an emergency several months earlier when she was pregnant. Another doctor was thought to have no understanding of his patient's anxiety about her baby:

'He's a very hard man. I took her in with the heat rash and he moaned at me because it had cost him five pounds because I'd called out an emergency doctor on the Saturday, But I can't change him or I'd lose my health visitor.'

The third doctor was accused of showing no interest in his patients even when they were seriously ill:

'When he came to see me, he looked drunk and he smoked. The baby was bringing up phlegm, but the doctor said it was nothing ...'

She said she had no confidence in his judgment since he had remained equally impassive a few months earlier when visiting a friend's baby:

'He came to see her and next day it (baby) died.'

There were also a handful of miscellaneous complaints including difficulties in understanding what a foreign doctor was saying, and receiving conflicting advice from their GP and clinic doctor.

Comment on general practitioners

The great majority of the young mothers in our sample had friendly relations with their GP and found him or her helpful. What emerges most strongly among this small proportion of young mothers who did not find their GP helpful, was the reasonable expectation that their GP should show interest and concern about them and their babies and should communicate this interest to them. In some of these examples, this interest appeared to them to be lacking, and if the concern was there, it was not being effectively communicated to the anxious young mother. A howling baby with a skin irritation may represent a medically trivial problem, one not very interesting for a doctor to treat. For a young mother, anxious and confused, this may seem a distressing episode that requires immediate attention. Possibly some conscientious but busy GPs could benefit from being reminded of this difference in perspective. However, this example also raises the question whether young mothers, and indeed patients generally (see, for example, Morell et al., 1980), might not be better advised in advance about the recognition of minor symptoms which do not justify alarm. Ignorance must lead to inappropriate use of services. This is another issue to which GPs need perhaps to devote more thought.

Health Visitors

We also asked our sample of teenage mothers about their relationship with health visitors. Nearly all (95%) had seen one between the time they got home with their baby and the initial interview, and of the small proportion who had not, one-third wished they had. Three women said they thought a health visitor might have been helpful in getting them rehoused by looking at what one described as the 'terrible' conditions they were living in with the baby, three others wanted to discuss various feeding problems, while three simply wanted someone to talk to. One of these had a baby who had died and she felt she needed more support than she was getting; one women spoke rather vaguely of how nice it would have been to have had someone to 'explain things'; and another, 19 years and married, remarked that she needed someone to discuss things with 'other than a man'.

We then asked the vast majority of the teenage mothers who had seen a health visitor whether they had found her helpful, and no less than 90% of these mothers said that they had, three-fifths describing her as very helpful. This section, however, dwells on the small proportion (9%) who told us that they had not found contact with their health visitor helpful. No differences in basic demographic characteristics were found between these women and the rest of the women who had had contact with a health visitor.

Non-communication

We asked the women who had not found their health visitor helpful, why this was. Nearly half this small group said such contact as they had had with a health visitor had, in their view, been a waste of time. They alleged they had been offered no advice or had simply been directed to the local clinic which they already knew about, or that the health visitor had simply repeated information they had already obtained from other, usually professional, sources. In many cases, however, the problem really seems to have been one of communication. They remarked that the health visitor was 'difficult to talk to', 'she never said anything', 'she didn't explain things', 'she didn't talk much', 'she didn't answer my questions', 'she didn't tell me anything'. One 17 year old mother said:

'*I* had to keep saying things because it was getting quiet—*she* wasn't saying anything.'

A 16 year old single mother said:

'she doesn't talk ... you have to do all the talking ... If I ask her anything she doesn't give an answer in a sentence, just says "yes" or "no" ...'

Poor advice

Nearly two-fifths of this small group of mothers complained of being given poor quality advice. By this they meant that it was too theoretical, irrelevant, negative, impossible to follow, or simply that it was different from advice

33

received from other sources—doctor, clinic, midwife or relative. They made the following remarks:

'They have never had babies so they don't know ... She said anything I was doing, I was doing wrong.'

'*I* know my baby but *they* just go by the book.'

'... she's in her late 50's and never had any children of her own ... said I wasn't capable of looking after him ... forever telling me things that were wrong with him ...'

'Every time I did something, she told me I was doing it wrong, but my sister said it was right ... They seem to go by the book but every baby's different.'

'She always came when we were doing things and gave us wrong advice ... she said "wake her up every 4 hours" and the Clinic told me to let her wake up when she wanted to. And she told me differently about feeding, from the Clinic ...'

'She keeps talking about the Clinic which is no good to me ... I can't get to the Clinic.'

One 18 year old single mother summed up various complaints about the quality of advice offered by observing:

'They've never had children of their own and so they haven't any experience to help you with any baby problems ... They didn't seem able to offer good advice.'

'Interfering'

The third substantial category of complaints centred round the notion that the health visitors were too 'bossy', 'nosey' or 'interfering'. One-fifth of the mothers in this group mentioned this. They made the following remarks:

'They're a load of busybodies ...'

'She's rather nosey ...'

'They want to know too much what your business is ... "who's the baby's father" is really nothing to do with them.'

'She's always poking her nose into my business and not taking any interest in the baby ... She's interested in things which I don't think concern her.'

'She was interfering ... I think I just got the wrong one.'

One 17 year old single mother went so far as to complain to her Family Practitioner Committee because her health visitor had insisted on seeing the baby when she called, when the young mother was out and the baby was in the care of a sister.

In addition, there was a group of miscellaneous complaints. Two or three women each said that their health visitor was 'too rushed' or had 'no time' to attend to their problems, that they had failed to obtain help with housing problems that had been promised, that there were personality problems—they simply did not 'hit it off' with the health visitor assigned to them—and in one case, that the health visitor had actually caused an accident to happen to the baby by too vigorous inspection, which resulted in the doctor having to be called.

Comment on health visitors

These criticisms of health visitors made by this small group of 45 teenage mothers are, of course, entirely based on their perception of events. Some of these criticisms may be unreasonable or unjustified. If the health visitor gives advice that is different from that given by a relative or another professional, it may still be the right and sensible advice to give. The other may be wrong. Even though the health visitor may not have had children herself, she may still know more about looking after babies than the young mothers. One 16 year old single girl objected:

'She keeps on at me about keeping on the pill ... she gets on my nerves.'

In this instance, the health visitor's preoccupation may have been entirely justified, though it is possible that the way her concern was expressed was counter-productive in this instance. Moreover, the health visitor who insisted on seeing the baby when the mother was out may have been acting commendably if she feared for the baby's welfare.

It is not necesary to take all these criticisms too literally. Some are clearly an expression of irritation that the health visitors were not always helping in the particular way the young mothers would like to be helped. Similar views were expressed about social workers as will be seen in the next section of this chapter. However, it does seem that there is a problem of communication affecting quite a number of health visitors in their relationships with teenage mothers and this may need some attention. Young mothers need more information and more reassurance than may sometimes be realised. They need to be encouraged to look after their babies the right way, rather than being criticised for looking after them the wrong way. And a few health visitors may exceed their brief and delve into a young mother's personal history in a way that causes resentment.

But overall it needs to be said that the criticisms made of health visitors were exceptional. The overwhelming majority of mothers stressed how very helpful and reassuring they had found their relations with this group of professionals.

Social workers

Whereas nearly all the teenage mothers had contact with GPs and health visitors, between coming home with their baby and the initial interview, very few (15%) had contact with social workers. Not surprisingly, the proportion who had seen a social worker was relativley high for younger women (35% of women aged under 17 compared with 13% of other women), for single women (30% cf 7%) and for working-class women (17% cf 7%).

Over half (54%) the women who had contact with social workers found them very helpful, while another 32% found them quite helpful. Only 11 (14%) of the teenage mothers who had contact with social workers expressed disappointment with them. Sometimes this was due to personal dislike or the feeling that the social worker was intrusive:

'I just don't like her. She was nosey. I can't explain really but I just don't like social workers. My mum didn't like them and I expect it rubbed off on me.'

'They're just nosey. They like to know too much. They ask too many questions. They want to know everything ...'

Other times this disappointment was due to the feeling that the social workers were not prepared to try to help the mothers in the particular way they wished to be helped:

'I wanted her to find me somewhere to live as I hadn't anywhere to go. She told me to talk to my mother. That's no good, I wanted a place of my own ...'

'When I was pregnant, because I had nowhere to live either, I had her, and she said I had to find somewhere myself or go into Bed and Breakfast, but I didn't want that ...'

'She's more interested in the father's name and address to try to get maintenance from him ... I don't want him to have anything to do with the baby ... so she wasn't very helpful.'

One woman thought the social worker's views dated and irritating:

'He's (the baby) very active. She keeps on about sedating him, which I don't want to do. She keeps coming round and making a nuisance of herself. Her ideas are very old fashioned.'

The other women had a variety of complaints. They mentioned that the social worker had only spoken to them briefly, or did not seem to know enough to help them. One social worker promised to call on the mother a second time, but never did so. One mother said, mysteriously, that until the social worker called, she was receiving eleven pounds dole money:

'but when she'd been, it went down to nine pounds a week. Well, it just went down.'

Another thought her own social worker compared unfavourably with her friend's social worker:

'My friend who is pregnant is well cared for by the social welfare ... Mine doesn't help me at all.'

Women who would have liked to have seen a social worker

There were, however, 31 (6%) women who did not see a social worker but would like to have done so. Three-fifths of these had a housing problem about which they wanted to consult:

'I want to move. I'm getting depressed. You can't put a baby outside. There are wild dogs around. The plaster is falling off the front wall. I've reported it and they won't do anything. I'm really getting depressed because I can't put the baby outside.'

'I don't get on with my Dad, and live on my own with him. I put my name on the council list and wondered if a social worker could speed it up a bit.'

Money, social security, marital problems and depression were other areas that led some women to want discussions with or help from social workers:

'I have been feeling down. I need to talk to someone. The health visitor thought it would be better to talk to a social worker about depression after the baby. My husband's a bit funny. He doesn't give me any money. I have to fork out my own money. We don't have any money some days for groceries. I have to borrow from friends. I have had to put her on cow's milk because I can't afford powdered milk. He only cares about his car. The health visitor thought I'd be better talking to a social worker but she didn't put me in touch with one.'

'I had trouble getting family allowances and any money for the baby ...'

'I don't know what I was entitled to and they could have helped me maybe.'

'A mixture of things ... helping me to get baby clothes ... and get L— into playschool.'

One woman who would have liked to have seen a social worker had been battered by her partner:

'Well, I used to live with the baby's father and he's trying to take me to court for her. So I'd have liked to have seen how I stand. I left him when I found I was pregnant, after living with him for two years. I felt, when I was pregnant, I needed some help because he beat me up when I was seven months' pregnant.'

Perhaps the saddest case of all was the West Indian nursing auxiliary who had been told that her baby had died prematurely because she smoked 40 cigarettes a day. She, however, blamed her GP for the death since she regarded the ante-natal care she had received as inadequate. Her partner had long since deserted her and she suffered from poor health and was depressed. She said she knew enough about birth control but did not like being on the pill:

'I just take it sometimes.'

She had seen only the GP whom she regarded as unsatisfactory, but would have liked to have consulted a midwife and health visitor as well as a social worker:

'I would have liked to have seen them all because I have gone through everything, and now nobody is interested in me because the baby died.'

Comment on social workers

Most of the teenage mothers who saw a social worker found this helpful. A relatively small number, however, who had serious problems to contend with, fell through the net and failed to find their way to the social services department. Since most of these women had seen a GP or a health visitor at some stage, it seems that these health professionals may sometimes be neglecting their opportunities for referring appropriate patients on to social workers. One young mother remarked how useful it would have been to have someone to turn to for advice whenever needed, and another said she would have liked to be able to talk to a social worker to help her 'to make more sensible choices about life'. Such support, especially for teenage mothers whose own parents are unable to provide it, may be an important social work function which, because of its unspecific nature, is often overlooked. Given that many of our young mothers were subject to severe economic, social or emotional stress, social workers in their counselling and advisory roles may have a greater contribution to make to the welfare of teenage mothers than some health professionals at present realise.

Baby clinics

At our first interview, we also asked the mothers whether they had taken their baby to a baby clinic for a check-up when the baby was well, and all but 13% of the mothers said they had done so. The proportion of non-attenders was relatively high among women from the lower social classes (18% compared with 11% of women from the middle and skilled manual classes) and among women who had had other children (25% compared

37

with 11% of women for whom the 'survey' baby was their first child). The women who had not attended any clinic said this was because they were too busy, that there seemed no reason to go because the baby was perfectly well, that the health visitor or doctor called on them at home so that clinic visits were not necessary, or that they had had a previous child and so knew enough without attending the clinic. A few women said they were now about to pay their first visit. One woman who didn't like attending clinics of any kind, said:

'It puts my blood pressure up, going to these places.'

We asked the vast majority (87%) of young mothers who had taken their babies to the clinics whether they found these visits helpful and more than three-quarters replied that they found them very helpful (33%) or fairly helpful (45%), which seems an encouraging vote of confidence in the services provided.

However, 89 women (20%) said they found their clinic visits not very helpful and we asked these women to tell us why they thought this, in case their complaints could provide guidelines for improving these services in some places.

The two most commonly voiced complaints were about the quality of the advice offered and the overcrowding of the clinics. Occasionally it seemed to the mothers, no advice at all was offered even when it was clearly needed. At other times the advice seemed inadequate, conflicting or dubious:

'Everything you asked them, they told you to ask your own doctor ...'

'I just have him weighed ... they said he was overweight but didn't tell you how to stop it. You're supposed to cope on your own.'

'The health visitor contradicts herself. She's not very helpful ... One week she tells me I'm overfeeding him, next week, she says I'm underfeeding him. I don't avoid her but if I can go away without seeing her, I do. I just have him weighed.'

'Everyone tells you different. You ring the health visitor and you see the doctor— they tell you different. The clinic tells you not to feed him too much and the doctor tells you to give him more—as much as he wants. So between them, you don't know where you are.'

'My sister had noticed that he'd got a hernia but when the doctor at the clinic examined him, he never noticed, and I had to ask him about it ...'

Others complained about the long queues waiting to be seen and as a consequence of this that the staff were too busy to give more than hurried attention to the babies:

'They like to see you quick and get on to the next one. They're too busy down there. I waited over an hour one time—I nearly had to go home without being seen because it was feeding time.'

'They were too busy ... they just examined him and that was it—"bye, bye". They said, make sure he's dried properly, but they never showed me how to ...'

'There's so many people there, you tend to get shoved, and they want to get you all over and done with quick.'

'Well you've sat waiting for an hour, and then sometimes they're not even there. I always manage to get her weighed. But if you want to see a doctor you have to wait hours. There's sometimes up to 50 waiting ...'

Several young mothers said they missed being able to 'chat' to the doctors and staff. Others remarked 'they don't talk to you', 'I'd like to talk a bit more', 'it's just in and out and no time to talk'.

A few women mentioned the fear of infection due to the fact that so many of the babies attending the clinic seemed to have colds or rashes or minor ailments. A few women complained that the clinic was housed in an unsuitable and inconvenient building, was not clean or properly organised. Several objected to the patronising attitudes they detected on the part of the staff, who sometimes treated the young mothers like children:

> 'They seem to be rather bossy ... they moaned and groaned, and it was just like being back at school the way they went on ...'

The reactions some of our mothers had to ante-natal clinics (see page 29) show that similar problems arise in the two types of clinic. There may be room for improvement in appointments systems, but the real problem in some baby clinics, of too many clients and too few staff, is unlikely to be solved unless more resources can be devoted to making them better staffed, better organised and less hectic places to visit.

IN CONCLUSION

The overwhelming majority of teenage mothers, never less than four-fifths, had positive things to say about their contacts with health and welfare professionals in the ante- and post-natal period. Only a minority of teenage mothers had complaints about one or other of the health and social services looked at in this chapter. Moreover, the proportion of teenage mothers who described their GP's and health visitors as 'not very helpful' was lower in this study than in Cartwright's 1975 study (Cartwright, 1979); the proportions in her study were 23% and 19%, respectively (unpublished data) compared with 12% and 9% in our investigation. So the relationships between young mothers and these two professional groups may have improved during the late 1970's.

Interestingly, there was little overlap between the women who were critical of their GP, women who were critical of their health visitor and those who were critical of their social worker. On the whole, young mothers who had problems with one group of professionals, got on well with the other groups. However, there was some overlap between the women who were critical of their health visitor and those who were critical of the baby clinic they visited. The proportion of the women who found their clinic visits not very helpful was 56% among women who were critical of their health visitor but only 16% among those who were not critical of their health visitor. No significant overlap was found between women who were dissatisfied with their ante-natal care and those who were dissatisfied with their post-natal care.

Despite this lack of overlap between women who had complaints about one or other of the health and social services, the actual criticisms of the different services were rather similar. The women were concerned about long waits for attention, lack of time to talk, lack of personal interest in their problems, conflicting advice from different professionals, lack of clear and adequate explanations and occasionally intrusiveness. They also sometimes said that the professionals did not seem able to help them in the way they thought they needed to be helped. But as this complaint tended to be raised in relation to their need for better housing, this was sometimes based on an exaggerated view of the powers of these professionals to obtain preferential housing for them.

5 Birth control and further childbearing

In chapter 2 we saw that one-fifth of the teenage women in our sample had used birth control around the time they became pregnant with their 'survey' baby while nearly two-fifths had not used birth control at that time because they wanted or at least didn't mind having a baby. The remaining two-fifths neither wanted to have a baby nor were using any method around the time they conceived. In this chapter, we look at the women's use of birth control after they had had their 'survey' baby, their plans about further childbearing and the extent to which they achieved their plans for the period between the interviews. But we start by looking at some of their sources of information about birth control.

Sources of information

We asked the teenage mothers in our sample whether or not they had received any information about birth control at school. More than two-thirds (70%) of them told us that they had had at least some sex education at school, but only half (51%) of our sample specifically said they had heard birth control discussed during lessons. The importance of early birth control education for girls who leave school at 16 and thereafter are lost to formal education, as nearly all our sample were, can be gauged by the fact that two-thirds (65%) of the teenage mothers we interviewed said they first had sex when they were aged 16 years or younger. Indeed, 9% of our sample told us that they first had sex when they were aged 14 years or younger. So, unless the schools can make provision for their pupils to receive effective birth control instruction in their early teens, it may come too late to prevent unintended pregnancy.

In fact, more than half (57%) of the women we interviewed said they had failed to use any method of birth control when they first had sexual intercourse; this proportion was higher for women who first had sex before they were aged 16 than for those who waited until they were 16 or older (65% compared with 53%). This would matter less if pregnancy had been intended. However, as we saw in chapter 2, more than half the women admitted that they had not intended to become pregnant with their 'survey' baby when they did.

Women who experienced contraceptive failure at the time they became pregnant with their 'survey' baby were relatively likely to have subsequently asked someone for advice or help about birth control; 41% had compared with 28% of those who were not practising contraception at that time. Altogether, 31% of the women said at the initial interview that they had asked someone for advice or help about birth control since becoming pregnant with their 'survey' baby. As can be seen from Table 5, three-fifths of these women had asked a doctor for advice or help about birth control, just over a fifth had asked either a health visitor, a midwife or a nurse and a similar proportion had asked a relative or a friend.

Table 5 People who gave advice or help about birth control

	People who women sought advice or help from	People who offered women advice or help
	%	%
A doctor	60	42
A health visitor	10	25
A nurse	7	12
A midwife	6	15
A social worker	1	2
Their mother/mother-in-law	9	5
Some other female relative	6	*
A friend	6	1
An unspecified person at:		
their family planning clinic	12	5
their hospital	4	19
Someone else	4	3
Number of women who sought or were offered advice or help (=100%)†	164	277

*Less than 0.5%.
†The percentages add up to more than 100 because some women mentioned more than one person.

At the initial interview, the women were also asked if they had been offered any advice or help about birth control since becoming pregnant with their 'survey' baby. Just over half (52%) of the women said they had, mostly from doctors, health visitors, midwives or nurses. The figures are again in Table 5.

Women who actively sought advice or help about birth control were more likely than those who were simply offered such advice or help, to have been told about specific methods of contraception (73% compared with 64%). The methods which were most frequently mentioned to both groups of women were the pill (to 66% and 56%, respectively) and the IUD (to 34% and 29%, respectively). Altogether two-thirds (68%) of the women had either sought or been offered advice or help about birth control since becoming pregnant with their 'survey' baby.

Current use of birth control at the initial interview

Seventy per cent of the women reported at the initial interview that they were currently using birth control. The proportion was higher for women who had a stable relationship with their 'survey' baby's father than for those who did not. Thus, it was higher for married women than for single women (75% compared with 60%) and among the single women, was higher for those who thought they would eventually marry their 'survey' baby's father than for those who thought otherwise (76% against 39%). The proportion currently using birth control also varied with social class; it was higher for middle-class women than for working-class ones (82%

against 67%). It did not, however, vary with age, ethnic background or the number of children the women had.

As previously mentioned, a fifth of the women became pregnant with their 'survey' baby while practising contraception. These women, despite experiencing a contraceptive failure, were relatively likely to be current users of birth control (81% compared with 67% of women who had not been using birth control around that time). Somewhat surprisingly no relationship was found between current use of birth control and intentions about or reactions to the 'survey' pregnancy.

As was to be expected, the proportion currently using birth control was also relatively high for those who had asked for advice or help about birth control since becoming pregnant with their 'survey' baby (82% compared with 64% of those who had not asked for such advice or help during that period). However, there was no difference between the women who were currently using birth control and those who were not, in the proportion who said they had had birth control lessons in school and in the proportion who said they had been offered advice or help about birth control since becoming pregnant with their 'survey' baby. Perhaps as Reid (1982) has argued, motivation to use information is of greater importance than easy access to it.

As far as methods of birth control are concerned, the data show that in general the women had progressed from using the less reliable or male methods to using the more reliable or female methods. The sheath and withdrawal were mentioned more often as the women's first method than as their current method. The pill and the IUD were mentioned more often as the women's current method than their first method, though the difference was not statistically significant for the pill. The figures are in Table 6.

Table 6   First and current methods of birth control

Method	First Method	Current method at initial interview
	%	%
Pill	44	48
Sheath	35	15
Withdrawal	12	1
IUD	1	6
Safe period	2	—
Chemicals on own	*	1
Cap	*	*
Other	*	1
None	9	30
Number of women (=100%)†	523	530

*Less than 0.5%
†Percentages add up to more than 100 because some women mentioned more than one method.

Hopes for further children at the initial interview

Three-quarters of the women said at the initial interview that they wanted further children; a tenth (9%) said they were uncertain about whether or not they wanted any more children while a sixth (16%) said they did not want any more children. Different follow-up questions were asked of these three groups of women. The latter group were asked to explain why they did not want any more children. Half (46%) said it was because they were satisfied with the present size and/or composition of their family:

'I wouldn't mind having more but I think two is the right size for a family.'

'I'm satisfied—well I've got one of each. If I'd had another girl I might have tried again for a boy.'

Two-fifths (38%) said the reason was financial:

'I couldn't afford any more children. I couldn't give to them what I could give to two.'

'I don't think we can afford another child. Well we're just managing now and another baby would break us financially.'

A quarter mentioned fear or dislike of pregnancy or childbirth or other health problems:

'It was hard having her. I had a bad time. I couldn't stand it again. I thought I was going to die.'

'I was advised not to have any more. In the hospital they said the baby took too much out of me and if I had another it would just wear me out completely.'

Other reasons mentioned included not being married (11%), wanting to work and go out (10%) and children being hard work (5%).

The women who were uncertain about whether or not they wanted any more children were asked to name the sort of things which might make them decide one way or the other about further children. The most common reply, given by a third (35%), was a change in their or their partner's financial and/or employment status:

'We're not paupers but we're not rich. So if we had more money I'd like to have more.'

'We couldn't afford to have any more children but if my husband got a better job or a rise then we might consider it.'

The next most frequent reply, given by a quarter (23%), was their current child(ren)'s age:

'Well, when he starts growing up I might want another baby.'

'I think when A— gets older I'll probably want another one. When I see other babies I'll probably want one.'

Also mentioned were a change in their housing situation (18%), a change in their marital status and/or their relationship with the 'survey' baby's father (15%) and their desire for a child of a particular sex (10%).

The remaining women, that is those who wanted further children, were asked, 'So, can you say about how many children you would like to have altogether?'. Half (52%) said they wanted two children, 29% said they wanted three children and 19% said they wanted four or more children. If the women who did not want any children are included in the analysis, the average intended family size was 2.5 children, which is somewhat lower than the average size of the women's family of origin (see chapter 1). Altogether, 72% of the women wanted a smaller family than the one they came from, 16% wanted a similar sized family to the one they came from and 12% wanted a larger family than the one they came from. However, women who came from large families were more likely than those who came from small ones to want three or more children; 43% of the women who had three or more siblings wanted three or more children in comparison with 34% of those who had less than three siblings.

The women who wanted further children were also asked 'How long a time would you like to have between (the 'survey' baby) and the next baby? A third (32%) said they wanted an interval of less than two years; half (47%) said they wanted an interval of between two and four years and a fifth (21%) said they wanted an interval of four or more years.

The proportion of all the women who wanted to have their next child within two years of their 'survey' baby's birth was higher for married than for single women. The relatively low proportion of single women who wanted another child during that time was probably due to many of them not having a stable relationship in which to have further children. Indeed, the proportion who wanted another child within two years of their 'survey' baby's birth was higher for single women who thought they would eventually marry their 'survey' baby's father than for single women who thought otherwise. The data are in Table 7 which also shows that women who had one child were more likely than those who had two or more to want their next child within two years of their 'survey' baby's birth.

The proportion who wanted to have their next child within two years of their 'survey' baby's birth also varied with the women's reactions to their 'survey' pregnancy; as can be seen from Table 7, it was relatively high for women who had positive feelings about that pregnancy. Somewhat surprisingly, there was no clear relationship between the women's feelings about the timing of their next child and their use of birth control. So to what extent did the women achieve their family building plans for the period between the two interviews?

Further childbearing

A quarter of the women became pregnant between the initial and follow-up interviews; 16% were pregnant at the time of the follow-up interview, 6% had a live birth and 4% had had a miscarriage, stillbirth or abortion. Five of these women (1% of the sample) had been pregnant more than once; four of the women who were pregnant at the time of the follow-up interview had also had a miscarriage and one woman had had two miscarriages.

The proportion of women who became pregnant between the two interviews did not vary with the number of children they already had but, as expected, was higher for married women than for single women. This can be seen in Table 7 which also shows that the proportion who became pregnant between the two interviews was relatively high for Asian women, for those who were initially pleased about their 'survey' pregnancy and for those who did not think about abortion or adoption in relation to their 'survey' baby.

At the initial interview women who described their housing as rather unsuitable for their present needs were not particularly likely to want another child within two years of their 'survey' baby's birth. However, as

45

Table 7 Some variations in family building intentions and practice

	Proportion who at the initial interview wanted another child within two years	Proportion who became pregnant between the two interviews	Number of women (= 100%)*
Marital status at initial interview:			
married	28%	29%	304
single—thinks will eventually marry their baby's father	22% ⎫		
	⎬ 15%	15%	150
single—thinks will not marry their baby's father	9% ⎭		
Number of children at initial interview:			
none	(73%)		11
one	26%	25% ⎫ †	391
two or more	1%	26% ⎭	65
Ethnic background:			
white Caucasian	24% ⎫	24%	414
Asian	11% ⎬ †	45%	22
West Indian	(25%) ⎭	(22%)	18
Initial reactions to their 'survey' pregnancy:			
pleased	28%	30%	226
mixed feelings	24%	19%	182
upset	6%	22%	45
Thought about abortion or adoption in relation to their 'survey' baby:			
yes	10%	15%	74
no	26%	26%	380
Housing described at initial interview as:			
very suitable	23% ⎫	20%	148
fairly suitable	23% ⎬ †	20%	145
rather unsuitable	23% ⎭	33%	153
Current method of birth control at initial interview:			
pill	23% ⎫	18%	214
IUD	21%	17%	29
sheath	23% ⎬ †	37%	76
other	(28%)	(44%)	16
none	25% ⎭	31%	133
Total sample	24%	25%	456

*As the base number relates to more than one set of percentages the minimum is quoted.
†Difference not significant.

can be seen from Table 7, a relatively high proportion of them became pregnant between the two interviews. Possibly some of the women who were living in unsatisfactory housing conditions at the initial interview subsequently decided to get pregnant again in the hope that this would improve their chances of getting a council flat or house of their own.

One group of women who were relatively unlikely to have had a pregnancy between the two interviews were those who mentioned the pill or the IUD at the initial interview as their current method of birth control.

Altogether, 47% of the women who at the initial interview wanted an interval of less than two years between the birth of their 'survey' baby and the birth of their next child became pregnant between the two interviews.

The proportion was 17% for the women who at the initial interview wanted to wait two or more years before having another child and 22% for the women who at that time either did not want any more children or were uncertain whether or not they did. Table 8 shows that the data about whether or not the women became pregnant between the two interviews was consistent with that about their family building plans for the period in three out of four instances.

Table 8   Hopes for further children at initial interview by whether or not became pregnant between the two interviews

Hopes for further children at initial interview	Became pregnant between the two interviews		All women
	Yes	No	
Preferred interval between 'survey' baby and			
next child:			
less than 2 years	11%	12%	23%
2 years or longer	8%	43%	51%
Does not want any more children	4%	13%	17%
Uncertain if wants any more children	2%	7%	9%
All women	25%	75%	N = 446

The women who became pregnant between the two interviews (with the exception of the five women who had had an abortion) were asked to say at the follow-up interview whether they had intended to become pregnant that time or not. Just over two-fifths (44%)—10% of all the women in the sample—said they had not. Disturbingly, the proportion who gave this response was higher for women with two or more children at the initial interview than for those with one child at that time (71% against 38%).

These women who became pregnant between the two interviews were also asked to say whether or not they had used birth control around the time they became pregnant. Over a quarter (29%) said they had. Putting the data about the pregnancies that occurred between the two interviews and that about the 'survey' pregnancies together showed, firstly, that 59% of the women had had at least one unintended pregnancy and secondly, that 40% of the women had become pregnant at least once while allegedly using some method of birth control.

Changes in use of birth control

The progression from the less reliable or male methods of birth control to the more reliable or female ones continued during the period between the two interviews. The proportion of women relying on the sheath around the time of the follow-up interview was lower than it had been around the time of the initial interview. Conversely, the proportion of women using the IUD around the time of the follow-up interview was higher than it had been around the time of the initial interview. (See Table 9 for the data).

The proportions who said they had ever used different methods of birth control are also shown in Table 9. Whereas the proportion who had ever used the sheath or withdrawal remained unchanged, the proportion who had ever used the pill or the IUD was higher at the follow-up interview than at the initial one.

Table 9 Changes in use of birth control

Method	Current method		Methods ever used	
	At initial interview	At follow-up interview*	At initial interview	At follow-up interview
	%	%	%	%
Pill	47	52	72	83
Sheath	17	9	59	58
IUD	6	12	7	14
Withdrawal	1	2	34	34
Safe period	—	1	6	8
Chemicals on own	1	1	6	8
Cap	†	1	2	2
Other	1	1	2	1
None	29	23	8	2
No. of women (= 100%)‡	453	382	454	453

*The women who were pregnant at the time of the follow-up were excluded from the analysis.
†Less than 0.5%.
‡Percentages add up to more than 100 because some women mentioned more than one method.

Changes in family building plans

To what extent did the women's views about further childbearing change between the two interviews? Table 10 shows that 85% of the women who said at the initial interview that they wanted further children either still felt that they wanted further children or were pregnant at the time of the follow-up interview. Concordance was, however, less good for the women who said at the initial interview either that they did not want any more children or that they were uncertain about whether or not they wanted any more children; at the follow-up interview 58% of the former still felt that they did not want any more children and 23% of the latter still felt that they were uncertain about whether or not they wanted any more children.

Table 10 Hopes for further children at the two interviews

Hopes for further children at follow-up interview	Hopes for further children at initial interview			
	Yes	Uncertain	No	All women
	%	%	%	%
Yes	68% ⎫ 85	32% ⎫ 45	24% ⎫ 38	58% ⎫ 74
Pregnant at follow-up interview	17% ⎭	13% ⎭	14% ⎭	16% ⎭
Uncertain	3	23	4	5
No	12	32	58	21
No. of women (= 100%)	342	40	74	456

Altogether, 75% of the women did not change their views about further childbearing between the two interviews; 14% had become more 'negative' between the two interviews about further childbearing and 11% had become more 'positive'.

Analysis showed that there was little change in average intended family size between the two interviews; it fell slightly from 2.5 children at the initial interview to 2.3 children at the follow-up one.

Summary

Only half the teenage mothers in our sample had had even rudimentary birth control education at school, and for some of these this had unfortunately not taken place until after they started having sex—not surprisingly, therefore more than half the women had not used any birth control at the beginning of their sexual careers, and, as we saw in chapter 2, more than half had not intended to become pregnant.

Birth control practice, however, improved with age. This may be because once a woman has had one or two children, she becomes, perhaps for the first time, really serious about avoiding further pregnancy. This certainly seemed to be the case with the young fathers in the sample (see chapter 11). It may be that for a very young person, it requires the experience of childbirth and constant childcare to establish the necessary degree of motivation. Certainly, by the time of our second interviews with the young mothers, when the 'survey' babies were some 15 months old, 85% declared that they now knew enough about birth control and over two-thirds said they were currently using a method. Nearly two-thirds of these women were now on the pill, and most of the rest divided between those who had an IUD and those who relied on the sheath. At the same time, one-quarter of the women were now, or had been within the last year, pregnant once more, and nearly half of these later pregnancies had also been unintended, so one has to conclude that contraceptive competence is a long, slow business that takes time, experience and a stable relationship to achieve.

6 Marital breakdown and battered mothers

Women marrying in their teens experience much higher rates of marriage breakdown than those marrying at later ages (Dunnell, 1979). Although the vast majority of married women in our sample considered themselves happily married—at both interviews around nine out of ten married women did so—a small number had separated from their husbands sometimes within months of getting married. The first part of this chapter describes the characteristics and experiences of this small group of women whose marriages had broken down. It is important to note that the total number of separated women in this study is too small to be able to make useful statistical comparisons with the rest of the sample. Thus, the comparisons that are made should be treated as tentative and suggestive only.

THE SEPARATED

At the time of our first interview we found that four women had already separated from their husbands. One year later, when we carried out our second interview, we discovered that another 14 had now separated. But of the original four separated women, two had now resumed their marriages. This suggests that the condition of being 'separated', at any rate at this youthful age, may not necessarily be a permanent one. Had we been able to conduct a third round of interviews, we might well have found that a few of these 16 separated women (5% of all the married women) were now reunited with their husbands while a further group had now separated, possibly drawn from the group of 28 women who told us at the second interview that they now got on worse with their partners than one year ago.

The first four to separate

Of the four women who were already separated from their husbands at our first interview, two were aged 18 and two 19. They had all previously been low paid and unskilled workers—two were canteen assistants, one a laundry sorter and one a mail order packer. Three women had experienced battering and one heavy drinking.

One woman had been going out with her husband for three years before they eventually married. He was a twenty five year old salesman. She was not pregnant at marriage, indeed she was having treatment for infertility, and wanted to have a baby as soon as possible. Her husband, however, was 'shocked' when he learned she was pregnant and soon turned to violence:

'He belted me when I was six months pregnant, so I walked out.'

She referred to their marriage as a 'disaster' and had considered having her baby adopted. She discussed this possibility with her sister, who strongly disapproved of the idea and dissuaded her. She was now back with her parents, siblings and nieces in her parents' council house. There were eight of them in a three bedroom terraced house and conditions were desperately cramped.

Another woman had married a nineteen year old plastic moulder within one month of starting to go out with him. At first all went well and they were keen to have a baby. On first suspecting she was pregnant, both were pleased. But then:

'It went wrong and he started hitting me.'

Moreover:

'He was still hitting me when he found out that I was pregnant, as if he didn't want him (the baby).'

They were evicted from their home and the violence grew worse. When she was four months' pregnant she decided to leave her husband:

'I wasn't going to risk the baby's life.'

She acquired a boyfriend and determined on divorce. Her husband had never seen the baby. Meanwhile she was back in the parental home with her three brothers and son. There were seven of them in all, sharing the four bedroom house, and she was hoping to find a council house of her own shortly.

The third case in which violence featured concerned a woman who had married a 17 year old timber worker. She had been going out with him for several months before they married, by which time she was pregnant. She had never intended to have a baby then. Although she had had both sex education and birth control instruction since the age of 14, she had not used any contraceptives:

'I just never expected to get caught.'

On realising she was pregnant, she sought an abortion, but later changed her mind about it. At this point her young husband turned violent:

'He started battering me up all the time . . . I just told him he had to leave and had to get a court injunction to keep him away from me and everything.'

Now she lived with her sister and her sister's three children in a council flat and was on the council waiting list.

In the fourth case, drink was seen as the main problem. An 18 year old taxi driver's daughter married a hard drinking 22 year old building labourer after going out with him for more than a year. She was pregnant when they married but said she had wanted to have a baby while her husband had mixed feelings about the matter:

'We were happy before, but as birth approached things got worse.'

She believed that while her husband was pleased to be a father:

'He doesn't want the responsibility of keeping her (the baby) and everything—that's why he left me.'

She had suffered from depression and nerves. She had appealed to the health visitor and social worker for help and advice but all they were able to do was put her in touch with the social security agencies. She and the baby were now back with her parents and three of her siblings in the family's three bedroom council house. Although she was seriously short of money and in debt, she felt happier than before, as she thought her status within the family had improved since she became a mother and her family were now more friendly and helpful.

It is difficult to generalise about these four women except in terms of their background as unskilled low paid teenagers. Two were pregnant on marriage but two were not. One married within a month of meeting her husband, while another waited as long as three years. Three wanted to have a baby, while one did not and initially sought an abortion. The husbands ranged in age from 17 to 25 years, but in all cases evidently came to resent the pregnancy and turned against their wives in the course of it. All the women had returned to live with members of their family, sometimes in grossly overcrowded conditions.

One year later, however, two of these women were found to be together again with their husbands. Two were still separated. The wives of the 25 year old and the 17 year old men were now back with their husbands and rehoused by their councils. The former remarked:

'He seems to have changed. He's not such an old grouch any more. He seems better tempered ... more cheerful, more settled, more helpful. He just seems different ...'

He even gave some help with domestic tasks and with the baby. The younger husband was said by his wife to now help with virtually all domestic tasks and to give a good deal of help with the baby as well. She remarked on the improvement in their lives resulting from being rehoused.

The woman whose husband had been a heavy drinker was still separated, and was now allowing her parents to adopt her baby since she felt she could not cope with it herself. She felt guilty about this and suffered from depression. She lived in a caravan, which she hated. Nevertheless, she was still pleased she had the baby when she did, even though, as she observed:

'My marriage split up. I gave my child away. I'm in debt. Bored. Depressed ...'

She was waiting for her divorce so that she could marry again and said she hoped to have another child in five year's time.

The wife of the 19 year old plastic moulder was still living in the parental house, though the situation at the time of the interview was somewhat confused as her parents had themselves just separated and moved out of the house with her brothers, leaving her with too much accommodation. Her boyfriend always came at weekends and she was now pregnant by him and hoping the council would rehouse them both in more compact accommodation. She hoped to have two more children eventually as she liked looking after children, and said she was now very happy.

One year later—fourteen more women separate

By the time of the second interview, 14 more women were found to have separated from their husbands. All but three of these were pregnant when they married, one woman with a previous baby, not the one that was the subject of this survey. The woman, who had been married longest, had been married since the spring of 1976—about four years before the separation occurred. Three women had been married about three years. However five women had married only in 1978 and five in 1979 so that their marriages had all lasted less than two and a half years. One woman had both married and separated in the year between the two interviews, so that her marriage had lasted only a matter of months. On average, these women had now been separated for nearly five months, actual periods of separation ranging from one to ten months.

Extreme youth was not a characteristic which marked out the separated mothers from the rest, since all but one had been aged 18 or 19 years at the time of the baby's birth, whereas one-fifth of the women in the rest of the married sample were younger than this. Their occupational profile seemed similar. They had worked mostly in semi-skilled clerical or unskilled jobs before marriage, as clerks, cashiers, print operatives, machinists, sales assistants, canteen workers and hairdressers. Four of these women had parents who were divorced or separated, and two more had fathers who had died during their childhood.

Only two women had been going out with their future husbands for less than six months before marriage. More than half said they had been going out with their husbands for more than 18 months, so 'marrying in haste and repenting at leisure' does not accurately describe their situation. Indeed, despite two-thirds of the women saying that money was a problem for them, all but two of the women had informed our interviewers the previous year that they considered their marriages to be quite or very happy. Either they were concealing the true state of affairs, or, once the novelty of husband and baby had worn off, deterioration set in quickly. More than half the separated women said their pregnancy had been unintended, and one-fifth had considered trying to obtain an abortion.

Depression and nerves

Almost twice as many of the separated as of the rest of the women in the sample said they had suffered from depression or nerves during the year between the two interviews (see chapter 8). Eleven of the 14 women who separated between the two interviews reported it and nearly all ascribed it to the stress of separation and the problems of caring for children single-handedly. In half the cases, the condition was said to be sufficiently severe to stop them doing the things they normally did. While one young mother said she had attempted to commit suicide others described their differing symptoms:

'I lost a lot of weight.'

'I feel right down in the dumps ... I keep bursting into tears.'

'I woke up one morning very depressed and it lasted about two months, and then I woke up and it was gone.'

However, two-thirds of these women had said they suffered from depression or nerves even at the time of our first interview one year previously, when their marriages were still seemingly intact, so their explanation of the underlying causes of this condition may not always be correct. It is at least possible that their depression was a cause of the marriage breakdown rather than its effect. So why had these 14 women separated from their husbands?

Reasons for separation

We asked the separated women at the second interview why they had separated. One man had run off with another woman and had never been back to see his wife or child. Another had turned out to be quite different from what his wife had expected, despite the fact that she had already once broken off relations with him before they married:

> 'He stole money from me, didn't pay bills, spent the money, wouldn't work ... I left him once before. We'd only been married for a month and I left him and I'm not going back this time.'

Five women said that battering played a part in the breakdown of their marriages, and this was usually associated with other problems such as drink, vicious temper, infidelity and financial irresponsibility:

> 'Adultery. Spent all my money. Drunk every night of the week. He knocked me about as well ... I just couldn't live with him again.'

> 'He ... threatened the children's lives ... I'm still trying to figure out how I got to meet him, let alone marry him ...!'

Three men were felt to be immature and inadequate as husbands, fathers and breadwinners. They could not fulfil the role expected of them by their wives:

> 'He just changed for some reason ... He was not giving me any help with the kids and we kept arguing about this. He packed the job in and there was no money coming in and he just didn't care. I said to him to go. I'm better off on my own ...'

> 'He's good for nothing. He was bone idle. He used to spend money in the pub rather than on the bairn ... He's 25 but very immature ...'

> 'It was after I had E— it just dwindled off. I don't think he wanted her. He turned more to his car and his job and came home late ... There weren't even great rows—he wouldn't argue.'

The relationships between the remaining couples seemed characterised by temperamental incompatibility, a category that of course overlaps with the other conditions described, and a lack of communication:

> 'We didn't get on ... We didn't like each other.'

> 'There was nothing there ... We were just living together.'

Youthfulness, inexperience and immaturity probably featured to some extent in all these marriage breakdowns. It is difficult to see why some of these women ever married in the first place since their husbands seemed to them so unequal to the role. Part of the explanation may be in the often considerable social and economic pressure exerted on working-class women to get and to remain married since marriage is generally seen as their best pathway to support, status and comparative affluence. In 1979, the gross median earnings of women were less than two-thirds of male earnings (CSO, 1980) and economic factors alone may persuade some women at least initially to welcome even a doubtful marriage rather than rely on their own more limited earnings capacity, particularly once they were pregnant. In addition to poverty, depression and unintended pregnancy probably were the factors that propelled several of these women into premature marriages, soon to be regretted. One woman who had experienced all these problems, commented:

'I have got no feelings left for him. I have no intention of going back to him. The only reason would be financial, to relieve the burden of bills ...'

Contact with father

The children remained only in intermittent contact with their fathers once the separation had occurred. At the time of the second interview, only three children had been visited by their fathers during the previous week. Five fathers had not seen their child for three months or more. Five had visited very occasionally. One baby had died as a result of a 'cot death' in the intervening year between the two interviews. Half the mothers thought the arrangements were adequate, only one saying she would have liked for the father to visit more often. Five mothers wanted the fathers to visit less often since they thought they simply upset the children to no purpose or because they thought the fathers had behaved too badly or proved themselves too unreliable to be allowed to take charge of the child for even a short while.

Only three of these 14 fathers contributed to their baby's upkeep. One had to be taken to court to obtain this and he reluctantly paid the mother £6.50 per week. The other two men paid £12 per week each. Just over half the mothers said money was a problem for them, but this was also true of nearly the same proportion of the other young mothers in the sample. Asked whether, despite everything, they were pleased they had had the baby when they did, nine mothers said yes. Half the young mothers had now acquired steady boyfriends and only three mothers said that they thought things were going not too well for them now. Nine women thought they had changed during the past year. They spoke of 'maturing' of being more 'grown up' and realistic and also of being tougher and more disillusioned:

'I'm harder now ... I'm not taking no nonsense from anybody.'

'I have become very independent, very suspicious of people. I don't trust them like I used to.'

Three women spoke of their relief that their husbands had now left them in peace:

'I'm not afraid of what he will do to me, or if he will come in or not, or if he will be drunk if he does.'

Comment on the separated

Recent studies by Richards (1981) and others suggest that most fathers eventually lose contact with their children if separation leads to divorce.

He takes the view that this is damaging to the children and that great efforts should be made to maintain parental visiting. Unfortunately, the interests of mothers and children in this situation may not necessarily be identical. The mothers may wish to put their broken marriage behind them as quickly as possible and cease to have to think about their former spouse. 'Such an approach', comments Richards, 'may be appropriate for the adults involved but two-thirds of all divorcing adults have children and their needs cannot be met so clearly'. He supports making joint custody the norm. The attitudes of the small group of separated, though not divorced, teenage mothers in this study suggest that there could be serious problems about joint custody, particularly in the absence of regular financial support from the fathers. The recent Report of the Law Commission (1981) recognised that 'the most serious problem faced by the majority of single parent families are caused by economic factors'. Where relations between the former partners were characterised by bitterness and resentment, it is not obvious what effects joint custody orders could have on the lives of the children involved. One-third of the separated teenage mothers in this study wished the fathers to visit less often than they actually did while only one woman would have welcomed more frequent visiting. Probably, as the Law Commission suggests, further research remains to be done in this area before any definite conclusions can be reached.

Perhaps one moral of this story for marriage and youth counsellors at a time when so many teenage marriages end in divorce is that it is unrealistic to expect marriages to survive if immaturity is combined with adverse social and economic conditions. Perhaps the now unfashionable Victorian middle class notion had something to be said for it after all—of waiting to get married and have children until a degree of real independence and a certain minimum standard of living has been attained. In the absence of such conditions, it is hardly surprising that some young wives and mothers find themselves back home with their parents with a child to support, within a short time of getting married.

BATTERED MOTHERS

It is disturbing to note that three of the four young mothers separated at the time of our first visit, and five of the 14 who had separated one year later said they had been the victims of violence on the part of their mostly still very young and immature husbands. This figure is a conservative one for two reasons. The incidence of battering may well have been higher within the group of women we were unable to trace and re-interview. More important, we did not ask any direct questions about battering. All the cases that came to light revealed themselves spontaneously and by chance in the course of discussing other aspects of these women's lives.

In addition to this group of eight young women whose experience of being battered was associated with marriage breakdown, another seven women in the rest of our sample also told us quite spontaneously, without being asked, that they too had suffered in this way.

Of the total group of 15 self-confessed battered teenage mothers, three described themselves as still married, while the other 12 said they were single or now separated. Four of these women were aged 16 or 17 years, four were 18 years, and seven were 19. Some details are given in the second part of this chapter of those we were able to follow up a year later who have not already been described in the 'separated' group.

One young battered mother was a single 16 year old woman, whose baby had been born prematurely and had to be placed in an incubator at birth. She lived with her parents and six siblings and nephews and nieces in an overcrowded council house. She had not intended to become pregnant at 15, but she had rejected her mothers' advice to have an abortion. Her 21 year old ex-boyfriend, who was unemployed and as far as she knew had never worked, said he would marry her but she refused because he habitually hit her, she explained:

'If he hit me when I was expecting, he would hit me now ...'

When we visited her one year later, we found the baby had had three spells in hospital with bronchitis and other problems. The young mother smoked as did the rest of her family. The father still visited his baby from time to time and she thought he had improved somewhat in character and temper. She now thought she would like to have more children if one day she should marry someone else.

The three 17 year olds in this group of battered mothers were all single. One lived with a 23 year old farm labourer who was still married to someone else. She alleged she wanted to take the pill but he had prevented her from doing so by threatening violence. When she became pregnant, her mother advised an abortion, but she left this too late and in retrospect was glad she had done so:

'He (the baby) gives me more to do. I have always wanted a baby to see what it was like.'

However, she also said:

'I get depressed more now—but that's not because of the baby, it's because of the fellow I'm with, and him beating me up. I'd like to get away but I know he'd only come after me and beat me up again. My mum is too near, he'd know where I was and bash her windows in, and things ...'

Asked what advice she would give to other pregnant teenagers, she observed:

'... if they were battered like me and made to stay in the house, they should try and get away somewhere where the man won't find them.'

When we visited one year later, we found the problem had been at least temporarily resolved as the man was now in prison. The young mother had acquired a new boyfriend and had left her old home to live in another part of the country. She was being treated for depression and worried about what would happen when the baby's father was released from prison:

'I think he will try to get custody of D— and he will beat me, and find me out here in W— ... I shall have to be careful ...'

Another 17 year old suffered from epilepsy. She said of her 27 year old unemployed boyfriend:

'He changed. At first he was happy about the baby, but then he started to knock me about. I don't know why.'

So her father forbade him to come to the house whereupon the young man threatened to obtain a court order to give him access to the baby.

When we visited again one year later, we found the baby had had one spell in hospital with croup. The young mother was being treated for depression. She was living with her parents and three siblings in their hugely overcrowded home. She slept in the sitting room while her baby slept in the grandparents' room. The baby's father now visited only occasionally. Money was a problem, though she now received more supplementary benefit than in the previous year. She did not receive any support from the baby's father:

'I don't want to get involved with him.'

Now that she had shaken him off she felt altogether happier and despite her circumstances said she thought life was now going well for her.

The other 17 year old was a waitress whose partner was a 20 year old painter and decorator. Before she was pregnant 'he kept beating me up'. Afterwards, he abandoned her. She returned to live with her parents and siblings and was now suing him for maintenance. She reflected:

'I wish I was working instead of staying at home all the time ...'

A nineteen year old Sikh woman, married to another Sikh who had had a technical education to the age of 20, started off her married life very happily:

'He helps me all the time and does everything I say.'

However, one year later the marriage had evidently deteriorated rapidly:

'He keeps shouting "do this and do that" ... If I don't do as he says he starts hitting me. I don't like that ... He gets so angry. He's really bad tempered.'

One explanation for this was that he was now unemployed and at home all day, and this was intolerable. They were running into debt and unable to pay their bills or their mortgage. She had had an abortion recently. She would like to have seen a social worker to discuss her husband's problems and her own but had not been able to make contact with one. She thought they would now have to sell their house.

Another 19 year old woman left her 19 year old boyfriend after living with him for two years and becoming pregnant by him. He was violent, 'beating up' his girlfriend when she was seven months pregnant, rarely worked, and was in trouble with the police. She did not believe he would ever change his ways despite his probation officer urging her to marry him. In the event, she married another man by whom she was now expecting a second baby and declared herself to be much happier.

The other 19 year old single woman had considered having her baby adopted, but then changed her mind. Her partner drank heavily:

'He'd just go on drinking, drinking, drinking ... He'd come home and shout and swear and even put his hand to me sometimes ... in front of my child.'

One year later, the baby had had a spell in hospital with a fracture, apparently due to falling downstairs. The mother had had episodes of depression, had been pregnant again but had had a miscarriage as a consequence of being battered by the man and he was now 'up on a charge of child destruction and grevious bodily harm'. She had left him and was hoping to start a new life for herself and the baby.

Summing-up

In addition to their youth, depression, unemployment, poverty and poor housing were features in the lives of most of the battered women we interviewed. This small group simply constituted the tip of an iceberg of misery and immaturity, haphazardly revealed. It is a sobering thought that despite their experiences, several of these women should nonetheless have concluded that things had worked out better than they anticipated when they first realised they were pregnant. One has to conclude from this that if expectations about life are very low indeed to start off with, then perhaps almost any slight alleviation of acute misery may ultimately produce some expressions of satisfaction.

7 Housing

Housing is usually a major preoccupation for young mothers, particularly for those, the vast majority in our sample, who are not at work and find themselves at home all day with a baby. At the time of our first visit, we found that nearly three-quarters lived in houses while nearly all the rest were in purpose-built flats and maisonettes. However, they were much less likely to live in detached houses and more likely to live in terraced ones and purpose built flats and maisonettes than do households nationally (OPCS, 1981b). This can be seen in Table 11 which also shows that they were much less likely to live in owner occupied housing and much more likely to live in council housing. Altogether, one-fifth of our sample lived in homes they or their parents owned or were buying on a mortgage, while three-fifths lived in houses or flats rented from the council. Most of the remainder lived in privately rented accommodation, while a few lived in institutions of various kinds.

Table 11   Housing comparisons with OPCS data

	Teenage mothers 1979	Great Britain 1979*
Type of accommodation:	%	%
detached house	2	17
semi-detached house	31	32
terraced house	38	29
purpose-built flat or maisonette	22†	15
converted flat or maisonette/rooms	5	6
other	2	1
Tenure:	%	%
owner occupied	21	52
rented from local authority	58	34‡
rented privately	13	11
other	8	4
Persons per room:	%	%
under 0.5	1	41
0.5 to 0.65	20	26
0.66 to 0.99	39	23
1 to 1.5	38	9
over 1.5	2	—
Total teenage mothers or households (= 100%)§	523	11,375

*Source OPCS (1981b)
†Includes only self-contained purpose built flats or maisonettes.
‡Includes homes rented from New Town authorities.
§As the table relates to more than one set of figures the minimum base number has been given.

Although the women in our sample tended to live in lower status housing, they were no worse off than households nationally in terms of the basic amenities that their homes contained. Around 90% of the women lived in households with their own bathroom and a similar proportion in households with their own inside toilet. Three-quarters of the women had homes with their own garden.

Nearly half the women (45%) were still living with parents or relatives at the initial interview and not in independent households of their own. Given that the women and their partners tended to come from larger than average-sized families (see chapters 1 and 11), it is not surprising that the homes of those women who still lived with their parents or other relatives were much more overcrowded than the homes of the women who had established independent households of their own; 65% of the former were living at a density of one or more persons per room compared with 21% of the latter. However, in comparison with households nationally, both groups of women were much more likely to be living in overcrowded conditions. Altogether the women in our sample were over four times as likely as households nationally to be living at a density of one or more persons per room. This can be seen in Table 11.

Satisfaction with housing

A third (34%) of the women thought their housing was very suitable for their present needs; another third (31%) thought it fairly suitable while another third (35%) thought it rather unsuitable. The proportion who thought their housing rather unsuitable for their present needs was relatively high for West Indian women (63% compared with 34% for other women) but did not vary with other basic demographic characteristics of the women. Not surprisingly, women who thought their housing rather unsuitable for their present needs tended to live in the poorest conditions. At the initial interview, they were relatively likely to be living in privately rented housing, in flats, maisonettes or rooms, in housing which lacked basic amenities and in overcrowded conditions. This can be seen in Table 12.

Table 12   Housing circumstances by satisfaction with housing and mobility

Proportion at initial interview:	Housing thought to be:		Number of times moved during past year:		
	very or fairly suitable	rather unsuitable	not at all	once or twice	three or more times
in privately rented housing	10%	19%	9%	16%	22%
in flats, maisonettes or rooms	19%	44%	21%	31%	52%
in housing which lacked:					
own bathroom	4%	16%	6%	7%	26%
own inside toilet	9%	16%	8%	11%	35%
own garden	16%	41%	18%	28%	45%
at a density of one or more persons per room	29%	60%	51%	29%	50%
Total number of women (=100%)*	335	183	248	245	30

*As the table relates to more than one set of figures the minimum base number has been given.

When the women who considered their housing rather unsuitable for their present needs were asked why this was, more than one-third mentioned serious overcrowding and lack of privacy, especially in relation to parents and siblings:

'It's too cramped. There's five of us in one bedroom at the moment. He has to sleep in his carry cot as I don't have enough room to put his proper cot up.'

'It's too crowded and very embarrassing at night as we share a bedroom with my sister.'

More than one-fifth complained about lack of hot water, inadequate plumbing or heating, and outside lavatories. In a few cases, the electric heating facilities were there but were far too expensive to use:

'We've got an outside toilet which we share with the next door neighbour. We haven't got a bathroom. The only form of hot water is an electric water heater.'

'We can't afford the electric bills ... We don't use the heating. All we just use is the oil heater we got off my dad.'

One-sixth mentioned that there were too many stairs to walk up with a baby, a problem often associated with lifts that did not work or were dangerous to use:

'We are on the third floor and if the lift breaks down I can't go out. I can't get the pram down the stairs.'

'The stairs—I have to make two or three trips if I've got shopping.'

Another sixth of the women, who considered their housing rather unsuitable, complained of persistent damp resulting in peeling wallpaper, crumbling plaster and endless colds for the family:

'It's damp and the walls are falling down upstairs.'

'It's too damp for the bairn. All the walls have gone black, the ceiling and everything.'

Other problems that were mentioned were noise that woke up the baby and resulted in sleeping problems for the family, the bad state of repair of the dwellings and the chaos resulting from repair works in progress, and a generally poor and dangerous environment characterised by vandalism, rampaging gangs of juveniles, and even night-time prowlers. Lack of a garden, inadequate or non-existent laundry drying facilities, long distance from shops, and infestation by vermin were all also cited by several women who considered their housing unsuitable:

'We get all the smell from the bins downstairs and the flues ... I've got nowhere to dry his things and when he's asleep during the day the other children on the verandah wake him up.'

'Well I had it fumigated three times for black cockroaches and I've found them in the babies cot.'

Many women mentioned more than one of the above problems.

The frequent movers

Just over half the women had moved during the year before the initial interview. Nearly two-fifths (38%) had moved once, a tenth had moved twice and 6% had moved three or more times. The women who had moved at least three times were no more likely than the women who had moved less often or not at all to perceive the place they were living in at the initial interview as rather unsatisfactory for their present needs. Their housing at the initial interview was no more overcrowded than that of the non-movers, though, at that time, as Table 12 shows, both these groups of women were more likely to be living at a density of one or more persons per room than the women who had moved just once or twice. In other ways, however, the housing situation of the frequent movers was less satisfactory than that of the women who had moved just once or twice or not at all. At the initial interview, as can be seen from Table 12, a disproportionate number of the frequent movers were living in privately rented housing, in flats, maisonettes or rooms and in housing which lacked basic amenities. We therefore took moving frequently as an important indicator of housing stress while recognising that there were other women whose housing situation was equally poor even though they had moved less often or not at all. One young woman, for example, who had moved house once only, was struggling to exist with her baby in a caravan without amenities, too exhausted even to embark on the ardous process of tracking down adequate housing.

Altogether, there were 32 women who had moved house three or more times during the period spanning their pregnancy and the birth of their baby. Two-thirds of these women were married, as in the rest of the sample, and nearly all the remainder were cohabiting. Three-quarters were aged between 18 and 19 years, while the rest were between 15 and 17 years, which was also a similar pattern to the rest of the sample. While most had moved house three or four times within 12 months, a handful had moved so frequently they could not clearly recall exactly how many times. One 18 year old single, cohabiting woman had lived in no less than seven different places within the year, with three periods in private, rented accommodation, two periods in 'squats', one period in 'bed-and-breakfast' accommodation, and finally into emergency 'short-term' housing. She and her boyfriend and baby hoped to be rehoused from here into permanent council housing.

Common pattern

The following sequence of events broadly represents the housing experience of most of these 32 women, though at each stage there are a few exceptions with slightly different experiences. Case histories quoted later will fill in the picture of the individual circumstances.

The majority of these teenagers started the year living in the parental home, usually a council house or flat, and usually together with several siblings. Their boyfriend would move in with them and they would then become pregnant if they were not already, and then get married, usually in that order. At this point, due to a quarrel, or to overcrowding leading to tension within the family, or fear of the council discovering unauthorised persons living in the property, the young couple would make their first move, most often to the young man's parents or other relatives or friends who had a little more space available. As the birth approached, there was quite a lot of pressure on the couple to move since there was usually growing tension here too after a few weeks or months of shared accommodation and facilities. On several occasions a degree of collusion was evident. The host family would write a letter 'evicting' the young couple. Although they were not literally intending to turn them out into the streets immediately, their continued presence was clearly a genuine and serious inconvenience in the longer term. The couple presented this communication to the council in the hope that this, together with the imminent birth of their baby, would give them some housing priority. The immediate result was to be moved into one or more 'bed-and-breakfast' establishments or other kinds of 'short-term' emergency housing of varying degrees of decrepitude and inconvenience, sometimes at a great distance from the young man's place of work. Once the baby arrived, one-quarter of these couples were moved into permanent council accommodation, usually a two bedroom flat, but the majority remained in temporary accommodation waiting and hoping for such an outcome.

Despite differences in detail, the housing experience of those who do not quite fit the pattern outlined above, was also one of insecurity, overcrowding, lack of privacy and family tension. Some of the problems they faced are illustrated with individual examples.

Case Histories

One young woman moved from the parental home because her mother disliked the young man she married. They moved in with his family:

> 'We thought if we could get thrown out of there, we would get a place, so we asked her (mother-in-law) to write an eviction note and make us homeless. The council said we had to wait like everyone else—"everyone's urgent, not just you"—so they put us into 'bed-and-breakfast' ... up eight flights of stairs, and I was pregnant.'

After repeated complaints to the council, they were moved into an alternative 'bed-and-breakfast' establishment in another area, which was slightly better. Finally, when the baby was born, they were moved into a two bedroom council flat, without a garden which they wanted, but having moved house four times in six months, they were glad to be able to settle down at last.

Another young couple moved from parents to grandparents when they married. But after the baby was born the grandparents asked them to leave as the baby's constant crying had become disturbing. They were moved into 'bed-and-breakfast' accommodation with a landlord who cut off their hot water supply:

> 'My husband called the emergency social worker and he rang this chap, but he just hung up on him, so my husband phoned the police. The police made him give us a kettle, but the next morning he slung us out, so we went back to the council.'

The council agreed to transfer them to a second 'bed-and-breakfast' establishment but this turned out to be so far away that the young couple preferred to separate and they went back to live with their respective parents for a few weeks. Then the council was able to offer them nearer and slightly better 'short-term' housing. They had their own bedroom in a house they shared with other couples, but had no hot water or garden. Nevertheless they regarded this as fairly suitable compared with their previous accommodation, and they expected to remain there for about nine months before being rehoused by the council in a flat of their own.

The youngest mother we interviewed was only 15 years. She had run away from her divorced father's home with her boyfriend, been picked up by the police and put into care in a children's home. From there she was transferred first into another children's home and then into a mother-and-baby home which housed ten mothers:

'My Dad came and saw it, and it was a mess, so he took me back home.'

From home, the girl, her baby and her boyfriend were moved in as 'boarders' with another family. They had a bedroom, but shared all other facilities including an outside WC. They were private tenants in furnished property and regarded this as the best they were likely to get in the foreseeable future.

An 18 year old married woman moved with her husband into a flat rented by a friend of his, which they shared with him. When he was evicted for non-payment of rent they had hastily to remove themselves to other friends. But after a while they caused great inconvenience here, so they informed the council that these friends were making them homeless:

'We had to go down to the council centre. We had to wait all day from 10.30 to 4.30 and there was nothing to eat and drink. Then they came down and put us into a hostel.'

Eventually, they were moved into a council flat of their own.

Sometimes a homeless couple make great demands not only on their parents but on their extended family as well. One 17 year old mother lived in a local authority adolescent unit. On marrying, she and her husband went to live with her husband's sister and her five children, but they 'didn't get on'. So they transferred to another sister, but once more they 'didn't get on' this time with the brother-in-law who 'chucked them out'. They then transferred themselves to a friend of the husband and her family, where this story repeated itself once more—'she asked me to go'. The young mother then applied to the council and was briefly put into 'a place for homeless mothers'. Finally, before the year was out, they were all moved into a two bedroom council house, having in fact moved five times within this period.

It is clear that sharing overcrowded accommodation with family or friends causes resentment, stress and sometimes aggression. It is certainly not conducive to feelings of family solidarity. Such episodes were almost universal within this group of young mothers.

Changes in housing—one year later

At the second interview, a higher proportion of the women (76%) were living in independent households of their own. Not surprisingly, therefore, a lower proportion of the women at the follow-up interview than at the initial one were living in households of five or more people (17% compared with 34%). There was, however, no significant change in the tenure or in the type of their accommodation or in the proportion living in housing with basic amenities or in the proportion who thought their housing was rather unsuitable for their present needs.

Altogether, two-fifths (41%) of the women we re-interviewed had moved during the year between the two interviews; nearly a third (30%) had moved once, 7% had moved twice and 4% had moved three or four times. So over the two year period covered by our survey all but a quarter of the women we re-interviewed had moved at least once. In fact 42% had moved once, 17% had moved twice, 8% had moved three times and 8% had moved four or more times.

Of the 18 women who moved three or four times during the year between the two interviews, four had been identified as frequent movers at the initial interview. Thus for a handful of women with young babies, moving house every few weeks or months seems to have become a way of life. However, the housing situation of the other 14 women in this new group of frequent movers had seemed relatively stable at the initial interview.

Of these 18 women, nine were married, four having married during the year between the two interviews; one woman had separated from her husband; and five of the single women had split off from their former boyfriends, the fathers of the 'survey' babies. Three single women were cohabiting, but two with new partners, so the altered marital and pseudo-marital status of more than half of these women had obviously contributed to their need for new housing.

One single woman, for example, had split up with her boyfriend with whom she had been cohabiting, and returned to her mother's council flat. In due course she met a new boyfriend and moved into an aunt's house in another town in order to be nearer him. Finally, she moved in with the new boyfriend. One married woman left her husband and also returned to live in the parental home. As three siblings were living at home it was seriously overcrowded so she moved from there into council 'bed-and-breakfast' accommodation. This proved so unsatisfactory that she returned to her parents and while there became reconciled with her husband. Both of them moved into a large, very damp unheated six room council house. This was described as:

'emergency accommodation—and the council will eventually find us a flat.'

In addition to changed circumstances relating to marital status, partner's job changes also resulted in the need to move house, as did further childbearing. Two of these 18 women had had further babies in the intervening year, and two were about to give birth again.

Discussion

Teenage mothers are heavily reliant on the public sector of housing. In recent years there has been a persistent decline in the availability of privately rented unfurnished tenancies (OPCS, 1981b) and few teenage mothers or their partners have sufficient resources to get a mortgage and buy a house of their own. At the time of the initial interview, when just over half of households in Great Britain lived in owner occupied property (OPCS, 1981b), just a tenth of the women in our sample were living in a home they or their partner owned.

This reliance on public sector housing occurs at a time when the supply of such housing is restricted in many areas. Thus, many teenage mothers

66

spend some time in temporary accommodation provided either by the council or their family or friends. The frequent movers in our sample, for example, tended to move in with any members of their family or friends who would accept them for a while. The support given by the extended family to young women at this stage of their lives is very striking. In due course these young women would be urged to move when the pressures resulting from their presence had become too severe for the host family to endure. There would then usually follow a period in 'bed-and-breakfast' or other 'short-term' housing. What is striking here is the lack of control the local authority housing departments seem able to exert over the quality of the accommodation provided. Some of the experiences quoted by these mothers suggest that unacceptably low standards seem to be tolerated by councils despite the fact that they provide some of these private landlords with a steady stream of customers and an assured income. There may be a good deal of regional variation resulting from varying local housing pressures, but it does seem that there is room for improvement in the supervision exercised by councils over the private accommodation they rent to house their homeless young people temporarily, including the provision of hot water and minimum standards of cleanliness and lighting. To place a pregnant woman in accommodation where there were eight flights of stairs to be climbed, as occurred in one instance, also seems unnecessarily careless. Moreover, the conditions prevailing in some council-owned 'short-term' accommodation seemed as poor as in the private sector.

At our first round of interviews we found the frequent house movers were a group who were seeking to establish a new and separate family unit. One year later the majority of the frequent house movers were found to be composed of those in the process of changing their marital or cohabiting partners, or having further children and needing more space. Whatever the reason for frequent house moves, the process tended to be similar. The people involved had to expect to spend some time in extremely low quality accommodation while awaiting a permanent home.

Another hazard of frequent house moving might be thought to be greater loss of contact with the health and social services than occurred in the rest of our sample that had had the benefit of more stable housing. Our group of frequent house movers, however, managed to maintain contact with these services very well, though there was some evidence that more of them would have liked greater contact with health visitors than managed to achieve this. It is probable, though, that this loss of contact did occur among those women we failed to trace since the problems our interviewers failed to overcome in obtaining their interviews may have been similar to those affecting the various social and medical services.

It may be unreasonable to expect that every teenager who becomes pregnant or changes her partner shall promptly be housed by the community ahead of those who have waited on the housing list for some time. A period in various kinds of short-term, temporary housing may be inevitable given the shortage of habitable public housing available. There is nevertheless a powerful case to be made for councils exercising closer supervision over this section of the housing market or seeking alternative means of providing less inadequate temporary accommodation within the public sector.

8 Depression or nerves

There is some evidence that teenagers are particularly at risk of experiencing depression after childbirth. In Clarke and Williams' (1979) study, for example, the proportion of mothers who were depressed six months after giving birth was highest for teenage women. But as Russell (1982) has pointed out, little is known about how teenage mothers fare psychologically over a longer period. In this chapter we look at the extent to which the women in our sample experienced depression or nerves between three and 15 months after the birth of their 'survey' baby. We also look at the support given by GPs to the teenage mothers in the sample who experienced this problem.

Who reported depression or nerves?

Just over two-fifths (43%) of the women reported that they had suffered from depression or nerves during the interval between the initial and follow-up interviews. As expected (see, for example, Brown and Harris, 1978), it was reported more often by working- than by middle-class women and related to this, by women without a GCE qualification than by those with one. Also relatively likely to report it were the small number of women who had separated from their husbands. Asian women, however, were relatively unlikely to report it. The figures are in Table 13. There was no variation in the proportion who reported depression or nerves with the age of the women or the number of children they had.

Table 13 also shows that the proportion who reported depression or nerves varied with the woman's childbearing history. The proportion was relatively high for women who had had a previous abortion, for women who became pregnant with their 'survey' baby while using birth control and for women who initially had mixed feelings or were upset about becoming pregnant with their 'survey' baby.

Women who appeared to lack material and social resources were also likely to report depression or nerves. As can be seen from Table 13, the proportion who reported it was relatively high for women who said they went short of things they needed, for women who described their housing as rather unsuitable for their present needs and for women who said they went out on average less than one evening a week.

Other groups of women who were likely to have reported depression or nerves included those who reported a poor relationship with their spouse and those who described their baby as rather difficult to look after. Again the figures are in Table 13.

Depression or nerves appeared, then, to be associated with a number of personal problems or social disadvantages, though it is unclear whether they were a cause or an effect of it. So what did the women who reported depression or nerves think had caused it?

Table 13   Factors associated with depression or nerves

	Proportion who suffered from depression or nerves between interviews	Number of women (=100%)
Classified as:		
middle-class	30%	79
working-class	47%	315
Had a GCE:		
yes	34%	91
no	45%	365
Marital status:		
single	45%	128
married	41%	312
separated	(75%)	16
Ethnic background:		
white Caucasian	45%	413
Asian	23%	22
West Indian	(37%)	19
Had an abortion before conceiving their 'survey' baby:		
yes	67%	21
no	42%	434
Used birth control around the time their 'survey' baby was conceived:		
yes	58%	90
no	40%	364
Initial reactions to their 'survey' pregnancy:		
pleased	38%	226
mixed feelings or upset	48%	227
Went short of things they needed:		
yes	58%	106
no	38%	349
Housing considered to be:		
very suitable	35%	152
fairly suitable	42%	165
rather unsuitable	51%	132
Number of times went out on average a week:		
never	56%	55
sometimes but less than once	49%	127
once	40%	143
twice or more often	35%	131
Marriage rated as:		
very happy	31%	173
quite happy	44%	105
not happy	75%	28
'Survey' baby described as:		
very or fairly easy to look after	41%	403
rather difficult to look after	58%	40
Total sample	43%	456

69

Perceived causes of depression or nerves

When the women who reported depression or nerves were asked to say what they thought had caused it, 30% mentioned their 'survey' baby:

'I think it's him (the baby). He doesn't sleep. Cries all day long. He only seems to need three hours' sleep.'

'The baby has been bothersome, what with his allergies and all the colds he picks up. All this made me feel inferior as a mother and I began to feel the chains around my neck. The baby wore me out.'

'The baby got on my nerves a bit when she was teething and ill and kept crying and I didn't know why she was crying. Things got on top of me. I took an overdose through it once.'

'It's the responsibility of having a baby at this age (17). You can't just think of yourself any more. You've got to consider the baby's welfare as well.'

The next most frequently perceived cause, by 27%, was their housing situation:

'It's the house. It just gets on my nerves. We can't get another one until they pull it down. It's damp. We've no hot water, no bath, and the toilet's outside. It's just this place . . .'

'Being in the flat. I don't like it up here. It's too high and dangerous for the children.'

'Living at home with my family. They just get on top of me sometimes.'

'We've had to move about so much. I was at my mother-in-law's, then my mother's, then a half-way house, then here . . .'

Twenty per cent mentioned their husband, the 'survey' baby's father:

'Sometimes my husband wants me to do things for him he could do himself when I'm doing something for the baby. It's like having two children in the house instead of one. That's why I feel depressed most of the time.'

'I've had a bad time with my boyfriend. He thumps me about. He has tantrums and loses his temper.'

'Cos my marriage split up. He left us in March this year to go to live with another woman and left me with the children. I wasn't very good at all. I was very depressed and I took an overdose.'

'My husband's in trouble with the police and we've had to go to court.'

Loneliness and/or isolation came fourth in this league table with 19% mentioning it as a cause of their depression or nerves:

'I don't see many people. I hardly ever go out and I suppose that's the cause of it. I hardly ever go out and mix. I'm lonely a lot of the time.'

'I am only 17 and you think there is nobody there. My friends just come when they have nowhere else to go. They don't ask me out. We haven't got the same interests. They just talk about boyfriends. They're not interested in children.'

Eighteen per cent mentioned money problems:

'Mostly because I've got a lot of bills and my husband's out of work at the moment.'

'I've got myself into debt, I keep buying things to cheer myself up and then forget to pay for them.'

Other perceived causes were other health problems (8%), pregnancy (7%), and problems with parents (6%). Eight per cent mentioned some other specific cause while 11% could give no specific reason for having had depression or nerves.

Severity of depression or nerves

In an attempt to find out how severely these women had suffered from depression or nerves we asked 'Has your depression or nerves stopped you from doing anything since we last saw you?'. Twenty-one per cent (9% of all the women) said it had. Of these 41 women, 23 said it had stopped them from going out and/or mixing with people:

'I didn't socialise half as much. I didn't go and see the neighbours. Just hid away in my own little world.'

'I don't go out very much. I don't go out socially. I just feel that everyone is looking at me and if I go into a pub I have to get out quick.'

'If anyone came to the door, I couldn't answer the door to them. I just couldn't face people.'

Fourteen said that their depression or nerves had stopped them from doing housework and five said it had stopped them from looking after the children as they otherwise would have:

'I wasn't as patient with the children. I didn't turn on them or anything, but whereas I used to take pride in keeping them clean and dressing them nice, I stopped. I had to pick myself up when other people started talking about it.'

'I couldn't be bothered to play with him (the baby). Well I'd just put him in his cot and leave him.'

Other things these 41 women stopped doing were caring about their appearance, having an interest in sex, looking after their husband/boyfriend and going to work. Although these 41 women exhibited similar basic demographic characteristics to the rest of the women who reported depression or nerves, a relatively high proportion of them thought that their depression or nerves had been caused by their housing situation (49% compared with 21% for other women).

Consultation with general practitioners

Although the average consultation rate for the period between the two interviews was higher for women who reported depression or nerves than for those who did not (the rates were 3.0 and 2.1, respectively), only a minority (36%) of the women who reported depression or nerves said they had consulted their GP about it. A fifth (19%) said they had consulted their GP once about their depression or nerves; 7% said twice, 6% said three or four times and 4% said five or more times.

A group of women who were relatively unlikely to have consulted their GP about their depression or nerves were those who reported social support at the initial interview; the proportion who had consulted was 31% for women who had said they got on with their mother very well (compared with 45% for other women), 26% for women who had said they received financial support from their parents (cf 43%) and 23% for women who had said they went out on average at least one evening a week (cf 48%).

Somewhat surprisingly, the proportion who had consulted their GP about their depression or nerves was similar for women who said their depression or nerves had stopped them from doing something and for those who said it had not. There was also no significant variation with the women's basic demographic characteristics but the proportion was higher for women who thought their depression or nerves had been caused by some other health problem than for women who perceived some other or no cause for it (63% compared with 34%).

When the women who had not consulted their GP about their depression or nerves were asked why this was, two-fifths (42%) said it was because they felt their GP could do nothing for them. It was something they had to get over themselves:

> 'I don't think there is anything they can do for anything like that. I know what was causing it— (her housing situation)—you have to get on with things like that.'

> 'I don't think he could do anything about it anyway. It's to do with your mind and that. It's like only yourself can cure it.'

A quarter (26%) said their depression or nerves had not been severe enough for them to consult their GP:

> 'I just knew they'd pass off. They were just slight. Like normal depressions everyone gets. Well you must get depressed sometimes. Like before a period you get depressed.'

> 'It's not important to see a doctor unless it's continuous. I don't feel like slashing my wrists or anything ...'

> 'I never felt that desperate. If I felt depressed I could talk to my mum or my husband. I just talked it out. I never go to doctors much. I don't like to bother them not unless it's serious.'

A fifth (19%) said they thought their GP would prescribe them drugs which they did not want to take:

> 'She'd only put me on tranquillisers—probably valium. I'd be no good to the baby on valium. So I sort of treat myself. I work it off around the flat or take W— to the park.'

> 'Because he'd put me straight away on pills and I can't stand taking medicines unless it is really essential. Medicines make you worse. My boyfriend was on pills for depression and they just made him worse.'

> 'They only give you tablets that you get hooked on. Once you've had them you have to have them forever.'

> 'I think if you go to your doctor he just gives you tranquillisers and leaves you to get on with it. I don't think they've much time to chat to you, to explain things to you.'

An eighth (12%) thought their GP would not be very sympathetic:

> 'To be honest, I don't think they'd sympathize. They'd give you tablets and say that's that. I've had to tell them about my problems with D— but they say you have to cope and that.'

> 'My doctor's not the sort of person you can talk to. I don't feel I can. He's a funny sort of doctor. He seems to talk to me as if I'm silly. I'd feel he'd laugh at me. I couldn't feel comfortable saying I've got a depression problem. I'd prefer to discuss it with a friend.'

Other reasons given for not consulting their GP were a lack of time (6%) and problems getting an appointment or to the surgery (3%). Fourteen per cent could give no specific reason for not consulting their GP.

Prescribed medicines

Of the women who had consulted their GP about their depression or nerves, 70% said they had been prescribed medicines or tablets. Eleven of these 49 women who said they were prescribed medicine reported that they did not take any of it or that they only took it once or twice. Four said this was because they did not want to become dependent on it:

'I don't believe in taking tablets. I didn't want to feel I had to depend on them. It's no good is it—you've got to get over it yourself and not depend on pills.'

'It was a coincidence. The night I collected them there was a programme on television that showed about them. So I didn't take them. I didn't want to be addicted to nothing.'

Another four said it was because they felt the medicine was not doing them any good:

'I took them for the first two nights and they didn't help me at all so I didn't bother to take them any more.'

'They used to make me feel sleepy. I took them once.'

Two said they did not feel the need to take medicine:

'I think it was psychological. Once I had them I found that I could sleep without them. I think it was the fact that they were there if I really needed it. Partly I was thinking that I wouldn't hear (the baby) if I took them.'

And one said:

'I took a couple as me and my husband were having a bad patch. He took the rest as an overdose. I didn't get a chance to take any more. Then I just got myself out of it.'

Further, of the women who had taken their prescribed medicine over two-fifths (42%) thought that it had not helped them. When asked why they thought this, five of these 16 women said it was because they had felt no better after taking the medicine. Four others said it had made them feel worse:

'They made me a lot worse. They were the sort of tablets that made you happier if you were happy and worse if you were feeling bad.'

'I was always tired and irritable.'

The remaining seven women made some other comment. Altogether, 55% of the women who had been prescribed medicine for their depression or nerves either said that they had not taken it more than once or twice, if at all, or thought that it had not helped them.

Other help and advice

The women who said they had consulted their GP about their depression or nerves were also asked to say whether or not their GP had given them any other help or advice about their depression or nerves. Nearly half (47%) said he or she had. So what other help or advice about depression or nerves did these women's GPs give? Half of these women said they had been helped or advised to make specific changes to their lives such as to go out more often, to find a job, to move, or to change their method of contraception:

'He told me to go out more and to do something to stop me sitting around doing nothing all day.'

'He told me to get a job but it's easier said than done.'

'He said it was because of the place we lived in. He gave me a letter for the council about our situation to help us get a house.'

'Told me to come off the pill, that's all.'

Nearly a third (30%) said they had been advised to stop worrying and/or to take life more easily:

'He said not to worry too much and that I should take things easier and stop trying to do too much in one go.'

'He just told me not to worry about things—but it does not help saying that, does it? They are my problems, not his.'

A quarter (24%) said their GP had given them sympathy and/or reassurance:

'She was there for me to go and talk about it. She's been a good listener and has had time to listen and has been sympathetic.'

'I talked to him. He was very good at chatting. I didn't feel that I was giving (my baby) as much love as I should. Just talking made me realise that I was.'

Others (15%) said they were advised to forget about their depression or nerves and/or that it would go away:

'The doctor said keep your mind off the depression and it will go away.'

'He just said it'll pass. When I told him (the baby) was getting me down, he just said he'll grow out of it and that I'd have to pull my socks up and wait until he grows out of it.'

And one women said her GP referred her to a hospital:

'He's sending me to the hospital this week. I started having imaginations. I thought the house was haunted and I got the vicar in. The vicar said it was all in my mind and told me to go to the doctor. And then his wife came the next day and she said the same so I went to the doctor. He said it would be a good thing to go to the hospital.'

Contact with other professionals

The proportion who had seen a health visitor, social worker or some other professional during the month before the follow-up interview did not vary between the women who reported depression or nerves and those who did not. Altogether, 32% had seen a health visitor. 5% a social worker and 3% some other professional. However, twice as many of the women who reported depression or nerves as of those who did not, said that during the month before the follow-up interview they would have liked to have seen a health visitor or a social worker or some other professional; the proportions were 22% and 10%, respectively.

Discussion

Altogether just over two-fifths of the women were found to have suffered from depression or nerves between the two interviews, which were approximately three and 15 months after the birth of their 'survey' baby. It is difficult to compare this proportion with that found in other studies because the incidence of depressive disorders seems to vary with the method of evaluation and the type of sample studied. Our proportion includes women who had suffered from depression or nerves of varying intensity; the assessment was not based on standardised clinical criteria but on the women's response to a straightforward question. It may, however, be an underestimate for the population studied; as previously mentioned, the women we were unable to retain in our sample over the whole period of the study were more socially deprived than those we were able to follow up so it is probable that a higher proportion of them had suffered from depression or nerves.

In this a study a third of the women who reported depression or nerves had sought help from their GP. In the main, his or her response was to prescribe medicines. Over half the women who were prescribed medicine, however, either did not take it more than once or twice, if at all, or thought that it had not helped them. Moreover, a fifth of the women who had not consulted their GP about their depression or nerves said this was because they thought he or she would prescribe them medicines which they did not want to take. In all, over a quarter (29%) of the women who reported depression or nerves expressed misgivings about taking medicines for it. Other studies (see for example, Cartwright and Anderson, 1981) have shown that people are becoming increasingly suspicious of medicines and reluctant to take them.

If women who are suffering from depression or nerves have misgivings about being prescribed medicines, what help do they hope to get when they consult a GP? In Ginsberg and Brown's study (1981) three-quarters of the women thought that talking about their depression and their problems was the best way they could be helped. However, few of the women in this study said their GP had given them time to talk and had listened sympathetically. GPs may feel that they have neither the time nor the inclination to deal with social and/or psychological problems. Moreover, they may convey some of this feeling to their patients; an eighth of the women who had not consulted their GP about their depression or nerves said this was because they thought he or she would not be very sympathetic. GPs could, of course, refer women suffering from depression or nerves to other professionals or agencies who were prepared to give time and listen sympathetically. Our data suggest that there may be a need for this.

9 Smoking

When we paid our second visit to our sample of teenage mothers in the autumn of 1980 we asked them whether they smoked, and those who said they did we questioned in some detail about their smoking habits and attitudes.

Of the 456 women we interviewed, only 132 (29%) had never smoked and this included all the 25 Asian women in the sample. Another 55 (12%) used to smoke but had now given up; 269 (59%) were current smokers. This is a much higher figure than for teenage women in general. In 1980, in Great Britain as a whole, 63% of teenage women had never or only occasionally smoked, 4% had given up, and only 32% were current smokers, as were 40% in the 20–24 age group (OPCS, 1981d).

Who smoked?

Smoking appeared to be associated with a number of problems or social disadvantages (see Table 14). The young mothers who smoked were more likely to come from a lower social class and from a larger family than those who did not, and they were less likely to have any educational qualifications. They were also less likely to be married, less likely to rate their marriages as very happy, and more likely to be living alone with their babies. They were more likely to have financial problems. They were also

Table 14   Some factors associated with smoking

	Current smokers	Former smokers	Non-smokers	All teenage mothers
Classified as social class I or II	11%	11%	23%	14%
Has 3 or more siblings	68%	59%	59%	64%
Has an eduational qualification	46%	53%	58%	50%
Marital status:	%	%	%	%
single	34	22	19	28
married	61	76	79	68
separated	5	2	2	4
Marriage considered to be very happy	50%	59%	65%	56%
Lives alone with her child(ren)	10%	4%	5%	8%
Finds money a problem	63%	57%	46%	55%
Has suffered from depression or nerves during the past year	47%	51%	30%	43%
Number of women (=100%)*	235	44	115	394

* As the table relates to more than one set of figures the minimum base number has been given.

more likely to have suffered from depression or nerves than the non-smokers in the sample. Furthermore it was disturbing to find that half of the women found to be pregnant again on this round of interviews smoked, and that more than one-fifth of them smoked heavily.

The former smokers

Of the 55 (12%) women in the sample who had now stopped smoking, 26 had done so before the baby was conceived, 17 during the time they were pregnant and 12 after the baby was born. We questioned the last two categories further about this. Of these 29 women, 18 said they gave up smoking at least partly for health reasons:

> '... bad for your health—causes bronchitis, lung cancer and all these things ...'

> 'Everyone said it was bad for me. I didn't feel well myself. I was waking up in the mornings feeling horrible—dry and sore.'

> 'I just thought it wouldn't do the baby any good, and if anything had happened when she was born I'd have blamed myself.'

Associated with this, nine women said smoking during pregnancy had made them feel sick or ill and they had given up then.

Most interesting perhaps from the point of view of social policy were the six women who had given up smoking because it had become too expensive for them:

> 'Too much money ... I've been looking at the price of baby clothes. If I gave up smoking I could buy a lot more ...'

> 'I couldn't afford it really, at 70p a packet ...'

Three women said their husbands disliked them smoking and one had even threatened to leave her if she did not give up, though she did not really believe he would do this. Eight women gave more than one reason for giving up smoking, while two gave no specific reasons.

Current smokers

Fourteen per cent of the women in our sample were heavy smokers who smoked more than 20 cigarettes a day. This is exactly double the national proportion of 7% for teenage women in general (OPCS,1981d). Another 30% of the women in our sample smoked between ten and 20 a day, and 15% smoked under ten a day.

Nearly all the smokers in our sample started smoking before the baby was born. Three-fifths said they had been advised to give up smoking during the past year, mostly by members of their family or household, though one-tenth of the smokers had been given this advice by doctors, in nearly all cases their own GP. Only four women had been given this advice by their health visitors. Nearly two-fifths of the smokers had in fact tried, unsuccessfully, to give up smoking in the previous year, but this was probably made more difficult for them by the fact that nearly three-quarters lived in households where there were other regular smokers, most often their partners. This was true of only half of the non-smokers. One woman said:

> 'I find I can't stop smoking if they are all smoking.'

While another one remarked:

'It would be hard. Everyone smokes, my mum and dad, and my friends ...'

Reflections on giving up smoking

We asked the smokers how they felt about giving up smoking and found that two-fifths felt they were so addicted to the habit that this was out of the question. Many of these women added that smoking was their only pleasure or the one thing that kept them sane:

'I couldn't face a day without cigarettes. That's all we've got now.'

'It's the only pleasure I've got. I'm in all day on my own so I get fed up and smoke.'

'It's the only interest I've got.'

Several young women remarked that for those who did not drink, smoking was the only alternative pleasure:

'I can't drink. It makes me feel sick. And I don't go out.'

'My husband goes out three times a week drinking with his mates—I don't go— smoking is my form of relaxation ...'

'My boyfriend has his pleasure. He drinks. The only pleasure I have is smoking.'

Several others added that smoking calmed their nerves and helped them cope with their children:

'I tried (giving up) for two months until L— started getting his back teeth, and it was either chucking him out of the window or going back to smoking.'

'If these two are getting on my nerves, I just light a fag and sit down and let them get on with it ...'

Several women linked smoking with boredom or thought of it as a substitute activity:

'It's just boredom really ...'

'They do help relieve boredom.'

'It's something to do ...'

'I smoke when I've got nothing to do.'

'Just something to pass the time away.'

One young women summed up succinctly the feeling lying behind all these views when she said:

'I haven't anything to give it up for ...'

Another opinion expressed by several of the smokers in this group was that if they gave up smoking they would eat more and put on weight. Others thought of cigarettes as a tonic that lifted their spirits:

'It works as a pick-me-up.'

'It's my little luxury.'

Only a handful of women even among this group of 'hardened' smokers challenged the message that smoking was unhealthy:

'I think all this business about cancer and heart disease is all a load of rubbish.'

One women said despondently:

'I don't care what I do to myself.'

Another women in this group showed that she recognised the health implications very vividly:

'You're only paying for your own grave.'

One women made an intriguing remark which is in line with other research in this field when she observed thoughtfully:

'It's the only thing I do myself, isn't it? I have to do things for the baby and for my husband, but smoking is about the only thing I can do for myself.'

Clarke et al (1982) in a study among American adolescents found that the non-smokers felt much more in control of their fate than the smokers and wondered whether smoking is a way of 'expressing outrage at the perceived loss of personal control in social contexts'. There are many hints of this in the remarks made by the smokers in our sample though few expressed the thought overtly.

In contrast to the 'hardened' smokers who had no intention of giving up or felt they were far too addicted to make this a realistic proposition, another group of smokers, just over one-third of all current smokers, expressed, sometimes rather wistfully, the desire to give up or to cut down and often recognised that smoking damaged their health, their baby's health or their purse, or all three:

'I'd love to give up but you have to go to a clinic and I don't know how to ...'

'... if I stopped smoking I could spend my money on the baby'

'Recently, I've been thinking of trying (to give up) mainly because it's too expensive, and I don't feel 100% fit so it might make me feel better ...'

'I'd like to but my husband smokes as well so it wouldn't be easy. It's getting too expensive and it's bad for the baby.'

'It's expensive and also it's dangerous with the baby because she goes for them and also it damages your health. I did give up, not long since but started again ...'

The third group, just under a quarter of the smokers, expressed no firm views either way. The phrase 'it doesn't bother me' was a common response here. Several in this group had convinced themselves that they could give up smoking without trouble if they were so inclined:

'I don't think it would bother me. I have stopped before—so I know I can give up.'

'I'd give up if I wanted to. It's only social.'

'If we are too hard up I don't smoke.'

'I could give up. I gave it up for a day once.'

Discussion

Young, mostly working-class, mothers are not an affluent group in society; a quarter of the women in our study were receiving supplementary benefit at the time of the follow-up interview. Any regular expenditure on smoking must make significant inroads on their incomes. Many of our respondents explained that they were trapped at home with their babies all day, lonely and isolated and with little to occupy them. Smoking functioned as a substitute activity and interest, and, as several observed, gave them 'something to do'. That smoking should be seen in this positive light by so many young mothers may be seen as a sad reflection on what society has to offer them. Perhaps a more generous provision of day nurseries for young children, and social clubs for young mothers, especially on housing estates, might help to mitigate the worst effects of the acute degree of social isolation that some of these women voiced, as might the wider availability of part-time work, for a higher proportion of the smokers (43%) than of non-smokers (32%) expressed a desire for such work.

It is also disturbing that half the women who were currently pregnant smoked, despite the fact that they all had at least one child already and should thus have been exposed to some smoking education and advice previously. This perhaps underlines the importance of undertaking effective anti-smoking education at a much earlier stage before the habit has been formed. This education of course needs to reach the young men as well as the young women, for, as we have seen, smoking is a family problem in as much as women who smoke are more likely to live in households in which smoking is the norm.

It is, nevertheless, encouraging to note that over one-third of the smokers had attempted to give it up or were favourably disposed towards doing so while one-eighth of the women in the sample had succeeded in giving up at an earlier stage. The health message had reached some of them and others realised that smoking was a waste of money. Putting up the price of cigarettes would obviously have the effect of reinforcing this message among the significant minority of women who have doubts about whether they should be smoking at all. Any additional revenue gathered by these means might well be spent in putting over the health message more forcefully since this may have already begun to show results, in that the proportion of teenage women who smoke has fallen since 1972 (OPCS, 1984a).

10 Reluctant mothers

At our second round of interviews, when the babies were aged about 15 months, we asked the teenage mothers whether, on balance, they were pleased they had had their baby when they did. All but 11% (47) said they were pleased, as one might have expected. Once a child has arrived and grown to toddler stage, it may require some quite powerful feelings of regret or antipathy for a young mother to be prepared to say that she is anything other than pleased. We decided, however, to investigate this dissenting 11% further because from the point of view of social policy they are perhaps the most interesting group. Why were they, unlike the vast majority of their fellows, not very pleased about having a baby while they were still teenagers?

Housing and money

Nearly two-fifths of these young mothers explained their negative feelings in terms of material shortages: inadequate housing, insufficient money, usually both these things.

Once the women were at home all day with the baby, as over two-thirds were, albeit unwillingly, for most (74%) wished to work at least part-time, the fact that they often lived in 'rough' areas began to depress them and they realised it would now be very difficult to escape from a depressing environment. These women were also often short of furniture, carpets, essential baby clothes and above all, 'spending money', a small amount of money to spend frivolously on non-essentials:

'... I used to waste money on sweets or going for a meal. Now none of that. Just enough money to pay bills and buy food ... I have to worry about our baby sitter and money. I wish I'd waited a little while. I wish I was married but not had S- so that I could have got the house sorted out ... I'd like to have given him (baby) a bit more ...'

'I should have waited till I got somewhere to live.'

Immaturity

The next largest group, more than one-third of these mothers, replied that they were simply too young and immature to have had children so early. In doing so, they felt they had missed out on an important stage of their lives:

'I didn't really live my life before I had him.'

'I think I'm missing out on being young ...'

'I wish I had waited another five years ... I feel I've missed out on my life—I can't enjoy myself with my friends.'

'I was too young and it's been hard ever since.'

Several explained what it was they thought they had missed out on. This included the freedom to experiment, try things out, follow their own inclinations and put their own lives first for a while:

'The freedom to do what I want.'

'I just can't get up and go anywhere ...'

'... I should have done more before having a baby—like enjoy myself.'

'You think if you hadn't had him you wouldn't have missed him—and think what you could be doing!'

All these women seemed to be asking for a breathing space between childhood and the assumption of adult responsibilities. By having a baby so young their life choices and chances had been drastically reduced and they felt they had allowed this precious interval to slip through their fingers. Now they were stuck.

There were also a few who wished they had passed their exams or obtained a professional qualification before being tied down with a baby:

'I still regret not being able to finish my training (nursing) ...'

'I didn't want to get pregnant then ... not at my age, having a baby at 16 ... I didn't really expect that, and I was going to college at the time and I couldn't do my exams ....'

'I'm studying for exams and it's difficult.'

Relations with partner

One quarter of these women regretted that they had not had enough time in which to get to know their partner better and achieve a stable and intimate relationship with him before starting a family, or alternatively that they had not had the time and opportunity to put an end to a hopeless and disruptive relationship:

'... I'd rather have been married or had a secure relationship with her father ... It's a mess like it is now.'

'... I wish I could turn the clock back. I wouldn't be with his father right now—most probably gone abroad to America or some place and gone to a hairdressing school. If I wasn't pregnant, I would have left him by now. I wouldn't have got tied down.'

'I would like to leave my husband but I've got nowhere to go now ... I've made my bed, I'll have to lie on it.'

'I thought once we got married everything would be OK but it didn't work out that way. I'm not with my husband any more. I feel very bitter ... it's not very pleasant having to take your husband to court ...'

Jobs

One quarter of these women mentioned lost job opportunities. They said they wished they could have worked, or worked longer, both for the experience, fun, independence and companionship, and for the often desperately needed money to provide a financial cushion for the first few years of being confined at home looking after the baby:

'I wish I could have kept my job as I had a good job ...'

'I think I could have done something, worked, saved money and got everything before I had a baby ...'

'I would have liked to have had more behind me financially and career wise ...'
'... I would rather have worked, got married and got a house before I had a baby ...'
'I had a job lined up ... they did not want me when I was pregnant because I would have been lifting things ...'

The wrong time to have a baby

Most of the young mothers in this group thought they had had the child too soon:

'Now that I've got her I wouldn't give her away. If I had my time again it would be nice to have her in a couple of years ...'
'I think I had her at the wrong time although I'm glad I've got her. I was so young ...'

One young woman, after observing that she should have waited till she was older before having a baby went on to say:

'Just staying in the house is boring, you don't see anyone or talk to anyone. You get depressed and you slouch around ... to look after him for three hours is enough for anyone ...'

And another young mother who likewise said she wished she had waited longer, reflected:

'I'm not so happy as I used to be ... I get very bad tempered very quickly with everyone ...'

She went on to say that what she really wanted was a full-time job to enable her to 'get out of the house all day—I'd like that.'

The most reluctant group

The social and economic deprivation some of these young and reluctant mothers experienced, partly as a result of the curtailment of their working lives, merges, in a small number of cases, into a recognition that they did not really want to have a baby at all, at any time:

'I'd just like to change my life completely ... I'd just like to have my own house all by myself and not have the baby. I'd be happy then. I'd like to have money ...'
'I just didn't want a child. I did when I was pregnant, but after I had him I regretted it. After I had the baby I realised I knew what I wanted to do with my life ... I don't know what to do about having J-. It's hard. I can't see my life being trodden on like this, being shut in the house all the time ...'
'I think we'd have been better off not having kids. We're both too self-centred.'

Thus within this group of 11% of 'dissenters', most women said not that they wished never to have children, but simply that they were too poor or poorly housed, or too young and immature, or had too uncertain or unsatisfactory a relationship with their partner, or had had too short an experience of independent, working life to have had a baby when they did, and most of these women said several of these things. However, a disproportionate number of the 'dissenters' did say that they wanted no further children; 34% did compared with 20% of other women. Altogether, the 'dissenters' were four times as likely as other women to want a single child family.

Factors associated with disaffection

Further analysis showed trends in the expected direction. The younger mothers were more disaffected than the older ones, the single more than those who had married before becoming pregnant. Those who had not intended to become pregnant, those who had suffered from depression or nerves and those who felt their job prospects had been affected by the pregnancy were also more disaffected than the rest. Women who had sought an abortion and women who had considered adoption were more disaffected than those who had not but in both cases the difference did not reach the level of statistical significance. Altogether those who were upset when they first realised they were pregnant were now more than five times as likely to belong to the disaffected group as those who were pleased. The figures are in Table 15.

Table 15.   Factors associated with disaffection

	Proportion disaffected	Number of women (= 100%)
Age at 'survey' baby's birth:		
under 17	21%	43
17	14%	77
18	10%	131
19	7%	195
Marital status:		
single	17%	145
married after conceiving 'survey' baby	10%	162
married before conceiving 'survey' baby	4%	137
Pregnancy intended:		
yes	6%	201
no	14%	237
Had suffered from depression or nerves between the two interviews:		
yes	16%	190
no	7%	256
Feels that job prospects have been affected by the pregnancy:		
yes	17%	99
no	9%	343
Had sought an abortion:		
yes	23% }*	22
no	10%	419
Had considered adoption:		
yes	24% }*	29
no	10%	416
Initial reaction to the pregnancy:		
pleased	5%	224
mixed feelings	14%	175
upset	27%	44
Total sample	11%	446

* Difference did not reach the level of statistical significance.

Resources

It is clear that the question of resources is crucial here. If every teenage pregnant girl could be certain of getting good housing before the birth of

84

her baby, a more substantial income, and convenient creche facilities for those seeking work, then most of the disaffected women would have been reasonably happy to have had their baby when they did. To some extent this is reassuring, even though the likelihood of these extra resources being made available is remote. At the same time, however, it is worth noting that while nearly one-third of these women had now found at least part-time work, many more of the women wanted to work, and some of these actually preferred to work full-time. The reasons they gave for wishing to work were the need for money, 'to get a break from the baby' and because they got 'fed up in the house all day'. One woman said she needed a change of scene because she 'got bored easily', another said she craved some adult companionship, another wished to work because her husband, who was at home, 'got on her nerves'. None of this suggests that remaining at home with a baby was seen as immensely satisfying or fulfilling by many of the teenage mothers in this group. One way of interpreting this might be to say that the teenagers were prepared to have babies at that age so long as they retained their freedom and did not need to spend too much time at home with only the baby for company. This attitude was summed up by the teenage mother who worked part-time as a cleaner who commented:

'If I had her all day she'd drive me up the wall.'

Many much older mothers might well feel similar sentiments, but for the very young mother whose contemporaries are mostly at a stage in their lives when social life is of central importance, the isolation of being alone all day with a baby is probably even more difficult to bear.

Discussion

The general picture that emerges is that of some nine out of ten teenage mothers being pleased with having their babies so young. One reason for this high index of satisfaction may be that those who would have been displeased were able, by use of birth control or abortion at an earlier stage, to contract out of the undesired responsibilities of premature motherhood. Given that around 35,000 teenagers have an abortion each year, (OPCS, 1982) and that many more than this seek contraceptive advice from GPs, clinics, and specialist orgainsations like Brook Advisory Centres for young people, this seems to be a realistic interpretation of what is going on, and a tribute to the work of the birth control and abortion law reform movements over many years, that have made these choices possible. The result of this self-selection process into motherhood is that the overwhelming majority of teenage women who do end up having babies, are pleased they did so when their babies have reached the toddler stage.

Whether they are less, equally or more pleased a few years later when the children are older, is another question, and one that we would have liked to have been in a position to answer had we been able to continue this study. Whether babies born to teenage mothers, whatever the attitudes of these mothers, do as well as babies born to more mature women, is also an interesting and important question (see, for example, Rothenberg and Vargo, 1981; Taylor et al, 1983; and Wolkind and Kruk, 1985), but, again, not one we are in a position to pronounce on, on the basis of this project.

There are, of course, all kinds of difficulties of definition inherent in coming to any conclusion about this. What do we mean by 'doing well'? Do we mean the number of 'A' levels they achieve and their subsequent careers, or do we mean living happily ever after in a council flat doing a part-time unskilled job? People will obviously hold widely differing views on this question.

Put another way, this study suggests that at least one in ten of teenage mothers with a toddler is not very pleased about having a baby so young. The real figure is almost certainly higher, for two reasons. The quarter of women we were unable to retain in our sample over the whole period of this research project were more socially deprived that those we were able to follow up, so it is probable that a higher proportion of these were disaffected. Moreover, there are almost certainly some women within our sample who did not wish to admit to any doubts about the wisdom of having a baby so young, for a variety or personal reasons including loyalty to the child. Over the country as a whole, this could mean that at any one time there are some 6,000–10,000 disaffected teenage mothers with very young children. Their disaffection is due to both social and economic, and to personal reasons. The former reasons could be changed, if, as a society, we decided to make the improvement of the social and economic status of teenage mothers a political priority. There are, of course many other groups competing for scarce resources and there is little sign that any government is likely to put teenage mothers on the top of its list of priorities. Some of the women, however, never wanted to be teenage mothers at all, even if they had been better housed and better off. They wanted to experience and enjoy their youth, and never got the chance to do this and now regret it. And there are also a few who did not particularly want babies at all, either now or later, as far as they could judge. With hindsight, it is clear that greater efforts should have been made to help these two groups to postpone motherhood, or even, in some cases, to avoid it altogether.

11 The young fathers

Much less attention has been given to young fathers than to young mothers. Yet this is an area where folklore abounds, often leading to expectations that young men in this situation will give little support to their partners and show little interest in their children, perhaps because they are scarcely more than children themselves. One young father in our sample summed up the latter view when he remarked:

'Weren't long ago we were children ourselves really. Now we've got one of our own.'

So why have there been relatively few studies of young fathers? One reason seems to be the 'mother centred bias in our culture' which, as Parke, et al (1980) observe is 'particularly acute for adolescent parents'. But there are also practical and financial reasons for not attempting to interview young fathers. They are less likely than young mothers to be at home during the day. They are more mobile, so that the costs of tracing and interviewing them tend to be higher. One per cent of our sample turned out to be in prison. Gaining contact with these men was by no means straightforward. There are potentially awkward problems about seeking to interview unmarried fathers who might wish to deny paternity, or keep it secret. Working-class men, as most of the men in our sample were, are not much given to discussing their attitudes and feelings, least of all with passing visitors. So, interviewing young working-class fathers is beset by all kinds of difficulties, which is why, given a choice, as the literature on young parents amply demonstrates, a captive audience of housebound young mothers looking after new babies, will always constitute an easier, cheaper, more accessible sample for time- and cost-conscious social scientists.

In this study we asked the partners of our teenage mothers about the pleasures and problems of fatherhood and of life with a teenage mother and baby. We thought this worth attempting because it is obviously preferable to ask people questions directly, rather than to rely on interpreting answers about their activities and reactions, given by others, as is so often done in the case of fathers.

This chapter, then, aims to take a snapshot of entry into family life from the father's angle of vision. In it we present our findings about the (mostly young) fathers' attitudes to marriage and family life at the time when the babies were aged about four to seven months and when the experience of fatherhood was still something of a novelty for most of the men.

Some characteristics of our sample

Nine out of ten of the men we interviewed were born in Britain. Ethnically, 91% were white Caucasians, 6% were Asians and 3% were West Indians. Four-fifths came from working-class families and two-thirds from families of four or more children. The average size of their family of origin was 4.6 children, which is comparatively large. Many (32%) had mothers who had been teenagers when they first had a child and 10% had mothers who were still in their thirties at the time of the interview. A fifth had parents whose marriage had ended in separation or divorce. Thus, the home backgrounds of the young fathers was similar to that of their parents, the teenage mothers.

Only a fifth of the men were teenagers when we interviewed them, a further two-thirds were aged between 20 and 25. Three were still at school or college while most of the rest (81%) had left school as soon as they were old enough. Over half (56%) had had no further education or training since leaving school and 12% were unemployed at the time of the interview, which was one-and-a-half times the rate for the men aged 16–24 in 1979 (OPCS 1981b). Most (87%) of the men had manual occupations. Just over half had married after their partner became pregnant. Altogether, four-fifths were married. Two-thirds lived in households that consisted of the man, his partner, and his child(ren). Eighteen per cent had children other than the 'survey' baby; a quarter of these men reported that not all their children had the same mother.

In chapter 1 we saw that the teenage men, men in unskilled jobs and men born in the West Indies were under-represented in our sample. There was also a relatively low proportion of men who were not pleased about becoming fathers then and who were not involved in baby care. It is likely, therefore, that the data we present in this chapter give a more favourable view of young fatherhood than is really justified.

Becoming a father: intentions and attitudes

A fifth of the men said they had been using birth control around the time their partner became pregnant; 11% had been relying on the pill, 6% on the sheath and 4% on some other method. However, about half these men admitted that they had not always used contraception while almost a fifth of them thought that they had not always used it correctly. Most of the rest ascribed their partner's pregnancy to choosing an unreliable method.

What of the vast majority of men who had not been using birth control around the time their partner conceived? Were they simply ignorant, were they careless or irresponsible, or did they intend to have a child at that time?

In fact, almost half these men who were not using birth control said this was because both they and their partner wanted a child, and in a few other instances at least one or other partner did so. Often the reason for wanting a baby at that time seemed to be connected with seeing pregnancy as a pathway to marriage:

'She wanted to get pregnant so we could get married.'

'She wanted a baby, and I wanted to settle down and get married.'

88

'We wanted to get married quickly. We knew her mum wouldn't let her, being just 16 ...'

In about a quarter of cases a mixture of ignorance, indifference, apathy, and timidity seemed to be at work. The ignorance may not be surprising. Only half the men had ever had any sex education at school and only a third had ever heard birth control discussed in lessons at school:

'I thought I'd get away with it and not get her pregnant.'

'We thought it would never happen.'

'We were a bit timid to go and ask anyone for help.'

The indifference may be more difficult to account for:

'I just didn't care. If she got caught, that was it. I didn't mind getting married.'

'She left home and left her pills behind so we didn't think about it.'

'It didn't bother us if she did, put it that way.'

An eighth had problems with or dislike of birth control devices:

'It wouldn't be the same if I was wearing something.'

'We took precautions at first but got so fed up.'

'She should take the pill because I don't like using the other thing.'

Others gave a variety of reasons for failure to use birth control, among which 'it just happened' was a common response.

It seems that a large number of these men were prepared to contemplate having a baby at that time even if not always with great enthusiasm. In response to another question just over half the men said they had intended their partner to become pregnant, though more of the married (60%) than of single men (28%) said this. And when asked about their initial reactions to the pregnancy 75% said they had been pleased while another 20% confessed to mixed feelings. Only 5% had been definitely upset by the news. As might be expected, more of the married (90%) than of the single men (66%) had been pleased about the pregnancy. Unexpectedly, however, more of the men than of their partners had been pleased about the pregnancy. Altogether, 60% of the men and their partners reported similar initial reactions. But among couples who reported different initial reactions, the man was the more positive in three out of four instances. This can be seen from Table 16.

Table 16 Men's initial reactions to the pregnancy by their partners' initial reactions

	Women's initial reactions:			
	pleased	mixed feelings	upset	Total sample
Men's initial reactions:				
pleased	48%	23%	4%	75%
mixed feelings	6%	11%	3%	20%
upset	2%	2%	1%	5%
Total sample	56%	36%	8%	N = 366

89

None of them considered adoption for their babies. Few (5%) of the men thought their partner ought to have an abortion and even fewer (4%) went as far as suggesting this to her, though this was sometimes because it did not occur to them in time:

'We didn't want the child and our parents didn't want it and we tried to forget it ... However, it was too late when we thought of it (abortion).'

The failure to suggest abortion as a solution to their 'problems' is not explained by the men's views on abortion. Half thought that in principle any woman who wanted an abortion should be able to obtain one. Only 10% disagreed with this. The remaining 40% thought abortion ought to be available where there was acceptable grounds for this. What these were varied from narrow medical indications to the widest social indications:

'If she is too young, or has no husband, or cannot support herself.'
'If the mother will be harmed herself.'
'If she knew the child was going to be subnormal or something.'

One man who gave a qualified reply nonetheless went on to explain:

'Only if the woman wants it. I don't think the man should have any say. It's the woman who's got to go through having the baby.'

Certainly, the majority of men could be described as having liberal views on this subject.

Life together

As previously mentioned, four-fifths of the men in our sample were married. Only four of these men said their marriage was unhappy and only eight more had mixed feelings about it. This is a remarkably high index of satisfaction with matrimony and, given the high rates of divorce for marriages where the bride is a teenager (Rimmer, 1981), it would be interesting to know how long this high level of satisfaction lasts:

'We just seem to do everything together. It's great.'
'We're ideally suited.'

Though there were a few clouds, even among those who claimed to be happy:

'The novelty has worn off a bit now. Before we went around and got on but now tempers fly a bit.'
'Somehow we get depressed with each other and the baby ... I get depressed with my job. It's so boring doing the same thing all the time.'

One man who admitted to being unhappy observed:

'I think it's the kids that's not making it very happy ... We're always having arguments about not having enough money, what debt we're in.'

And another:

'I don't like married life. I'm tied down with it 'cos we have the kids.'

Also previously mentioned was the fact that half of the married men in our sample had married while their partner was pregnant. Nearly three-fifths of these men said the pregnancy was the main reason for getting married at that time. However, all but three also said they would have got married to their wife anyway at some time in the future.

Nearly all (91%) of the men who remained single had talked about the question of marriage at some time with their partners. Reactions varied:

'I did when I found out she was pregnant, but she turned me down and said to wait until the baby was born. I respect her for that and as it's turned out she was right.'

'We'd rather wait first to see if we can live together and then maybe get married.'

Just over two-fifths had also discussed the question of marriage with their parents or others. Most thought they would get married to their partners before long. Only 14% said definitely not, the reasons varying from not being in love, being happy as they were, having no money or jobs, to the girl having gone off with someone else. Just one man was against the idea of marriage on principle.

A high proportion of young fathers, single as well as married, claimed to have helped their partner with domestic tasks the previous week. Three-quarters had helped with shopping and three-fifths with cleaning, washing up, cooking and household repairs. Fewer men, though, reported assisting with making the beds (51%), washing (30%) or ironing (20%). Only some 5% of men who were in a position to do so, said they had not helped with anything.

Altogether, a third of the men thought their relationship with their partner had improved since she became pregnant:

'It's brought us closer together.'

'I feel we're more of a family.'

Some of these men did, however, mention problems:

'We had to move in with her mother during some months of the pregnancy. The pressure told on her, but then things got back OK again.'

'I wanted to get married in a hurry. She felt she was being rushed. Then I felt I wasn't wanted. Then it got better.'

Half the men thought their relationship with their partner had not changed since she became pregnant. Only 7% thought it had deteriorated:

'We argue a bit more.'

The remaining 7% made some other comment.

Birth Control

After the baby was born the men appeared to be much more careful about their birth control practices. Whereas 80% had not used contraception around the time their partner became pregnant, 80% had adopted a method after the baby had arrived. The methods of birth control the men were relying on around the time of the interview are shown in the last column of Table 17.

Table 17 also shows the methods of birth control the men had used initially. Comparison of the men's initial methods of birth control with

Table 17 Use of birth control

Method	First method	Current method
	%	%
Sheath	59	23
Pill	22	53
Withdrawal	15	1
Safe period	1	1
Chemicals	1	1
Cap	—	1
IUD	1	6
Others	—	—
No method	4	20
Number of fathers (= 100%)*	356	354

*Percentages in some cases add up to more than 100 because some had used more than one method.

their current methods showed that in general the men had progressed from relying on the less reliable or male methods to relying on the more reliable or female methods. The sheath and withdrawal were mentioned more often as a first than as a current method; conversely, the pill and the IUD were mentioned more often as a current than as a first method. In chapter 5 a similar pattern of birth control use was seen with the women.

This more effective use of contraception once they had a baby had developed despite the fact that only 12% of the men had asked or been asked by a professional since the baby's birth whether they would like any further information about the subject. It seems that, having had one baby, most were now determined not to have another in a hurry. In fact, 12% did not want any more children, and 62% of those who did, wanted to wait two years or more for their next child. Altogether, 64% of the men wanted one or two children, 23% wanted three children and 13% wanted four or more children. Their average intended family size was 2.5 children which was barely half the average size of their family of origin.

Father and baby

Almost all (98%) of the fathers said they felt responsible for the baby's welfare, in many cases simply because it was their baby:

'He's my son and I'm his father.'

In a few cases their feelings of personal responsibility was linked to particular experiences of their own, both positive and negative:

'My parents have been good to me and I hope that I can teach him properly and not shirk his responsibilities.'

'I didn't want to leave her without a dad because I know how it feels. I was brought up just by my mum. I know how the baby feels and I didn't want that to happen.'

Several fathers said they changed their life-style in order to take account of the baby's arrival:

'I go out to work to support her. I've cut down my drinking and I don't smoke so much.'

Nearly half the men specifically mentioned their role as breadwinners as an aspect of their feelings of responsibility for their child.

Virtually all (97%) of the fathers claimed to have helped look after their baby at least occasionally. The most frequently reported task seemed to be feeding the baby and the least frequently, bathing the baby. This can be seen from Table 18. Altogether, 52% of the men thought their baby was very easy to look after and a further 43% thought he or she was fairly easy to look after. Only 5% thought their baby was rather difficult to look after.

Table 18   What the fathers had done for their babies

	Proportion who had ever:
	%
Fed him/her	96
Changed his/her nappy	81
Looked after him/her while his/her mother has been out for an hour or more	81
Dressed him/her	78
Got up to him/her at night	76
Taken him/her out	56
Bathed him/her	48
Number of fathers (=100%)*	329

*As the table relates to more than one set of figures the minimum base number has been given.

They were asked what they enjoyed most about fatherhood. Watching the child grow and develop was often mentioned—'more interesting than telly' as one father observed, as was the sheer fact of having a child:

'You've got something that belongs to you.'

Another factor was having something that was admired by others, even strangers on the street. A few men, however, were indifferent:

'Nothing really ... I don't think about it all that much at the moment, honestly.'

Noise and changing nappies were often mentioned as the most disliked aspects of fatherhood. Other dislikes included the problems of taking a pram everywhere, and the dependence on babysitters which made it difficult to have much social life. Several also missed their previous freedom and 'not being able to go drinking with the boys'. Nearly three-fifths of the men, however, could not think of anything they disliked about being a father.

Half the single men did not have their child living with them. Most, though, had seen their child at least once, and often several times, during the week prior to the interview. Of the ten men who had not seen their child during this period, four reported that it was at least a month since they had seen their child and one that he had never set eyes on his child. These five men seemed, to varying degrees, upset by this lack of contact. For example:

'I don't like it at all. She's my kid. I'd like to see her.'

In all, 70% of the men who were not living with their children declared that they would like to see them more often.

Work, money and social life

Had becoming a father so young affected their job prospects? Only 17% thought so, but not all these regarded the effect as entirely negative. In fact a third of them thought their prospects had been improved:

'Given me some motivation, something to work for.'

Most of the rest of this group, however, felt that the effects were adverse in terms of mobility and learning skills:

'Now you're stuck ... I can't look round now, I've got to keep working.'

'I'm not very free to do the things I wanted to do.'

'I had intended to continue what I was doing but left a "good" technician's job to earn more money ... there's so much scope in a technician's work, and you never stop learning—whereas the work I'm doing now, there's nothing more to learn ... now possibly might have trouble getting back being a technician.'

Despite this, only 7% were unhappy with their current jobs while another 16% had mixed feelings.

The men's earnings were relatively low. In 1979 the average net weekly wage for men in full-time employment was £70 per week (OPCS, 1981b). In our sample two-thirds of the men took home less than this amount; their average earnings after deductions were £62 per week. Not surprisingly, more than half of all the men said money was a problem for them, in some cases acutely so:

'I'm always short of grub and that.'

'I owe money to people.'

About one-sixth of all men thought they were actually worse off than their contemporaries:

'We must be the worst dressed couple around.'

This was often associated with the expense of having a baby:

'A lot of people my age aren't married, haven't got a family, so have just themselves to support.'   .

On the other hand, just over a fifth of the men thought they were better off than their contemporaries, many of whom were unemployed or living on very low wages.

Turning to financial assistance, three-fifths of the unmarried men claimed to give their partners money regularly, and a few more gave money intermittently. Of the men who gave regularly, half gave less that ten pounds per week and a third 15 pounds or more a week. One man explained why he did not give regular financial assistance:

'I'm putting my money away for when we get married and I do buy clothes for the baby. She gets money from the Social so I don't need to give her any.'

Money problems obviously affected social life. Although the men tended to go out more often than their partners—on average 1.5 evenings per week compared with 1.1 evenings for their partners—the majority (61%) went out less than before the baby was born. Three-quarters of the men who now went out less often than before were content to accept the situation, finding their domestic preoccupations and hobbies an agreeable substitute for their previous social life, much of which took place in pubs:

'Doesn't bother me. Whereas before the wife would go out numerous times, now we've got an activity in the baby and an interest at night when we're all at home.'

'Not bothered. When we did go out, it was just sitting in the same pub with the same people. We don't miss it that much.'

'I prefer it 'cos I like home life. It's better than boozing all the time.'

'I don't mind 'cos I have a lot of home hobbies now and my time is taken up by them.'

It seems that in the past many young men often went out simply because they had little privacy at home in which to conduct their social life. This is not surprising since, as previously mentioned, two-thirds had three or more siblings. So their previous social life was often not greatly regretted. But this was not universally true. One-sixth of the men who went out less often did have complaints:

'It affects me 'cos if I want to go out I have to suffer and stay in, or have an argument with the wife when I get home.'

'I feel bad about it. If you are at work all day you want to get out in the evening.'

Some reflections

Looking back over their experience of fatherhood, 59% thought things had worked out better than they had expected when they found out their partner was pregnant. Only 8% thought things had gone worse than expected. The reasons given for this deterioration were what they regarded as external factors—interfering social workers, tiresome in-laws, the appearance of another woman on the scene, or adverse economic factors:

'With me not being in work our marriage is breaking up. She says she's going to leave me soon if I don't get a job, and get her mother to look after the baby and go out to work herself.'

Where things had gone well, it was because the man now earned more money than he had expected to, the couple had managed to obtain a house more quickly than anticipated, the relationship with parents and in-laws had improved, the couple had got on together much better than expected, and problems generally had proved less intractable than at first feared:

'I thought there'd be more things to it—having the baby would make things complicated—but it doesn't.'

Nearly three-fifths of the men thought they had changed since becoming a father, and in virtually all cases for the better. They felt they were no longer simply youths out for a good time, but mature and responsible citizens:

'I didn't used to give a damn about anything—but now I have to.'

'It made me older.'

95

'Quietened down, less of a hooligan.'

'Don't drink as much. Take pride in myself ... Have to keep hold of money these days 'cos I need to look after my wife and kid.'

'I haven't got a police record or anything. I'm glad I got married early. It's made me settle down.'

Similarly, nearly two-thirds of the men thought their partner had changed since becoming a mother. Becoming more mature was again a common observation:

'She's become more of a woman. She's got responsibility which she didn't have before, like having a baby to look after. And she's got to watch where the money goes, work out the shopping, pay the bills, which she didn't have to do before. She's become more mature and responsible, having to do the housework, things like that.'

However, not all the changes were approved of; 28% of the men who thought their partner had changed thought she had changed for the worse. Some women were felt to be more tired, more preoccupied, more moody, more fraught, and less good tempered, another aspect perhaps of the impact of their new responsibilities:

'More possessive ... she likes me stopping in with the baby. More niggly over small things. She makes an issue of things that don't really matter. Very moody. I think she feels tied down as well.

'She used to be really easy going but now can lose her temper at the slightest things.'

All but 13% of the men thought their life was going well for them, although half the men said they wished to change some parts of it. Another 7% said they wished to change many parts of their life. What this often meant was better housing, more pay, a more agreeable job, and more social life. Some regretted that they had not saved more money before the arrival of the baby and thus got off to a better and more comfortable start to their married life.

Altogether the men expressed a high degree of satisfaction with life. However, they were not as satisfied with their lives as their partners were with theirs. As can be seen from Table 19 the men were less likely than their partners to say that things had worked out better than they had expected, that their life was going very well and that they wanted their life to continue in much the same way.

Table 19 Fathers and mothers assessments of life satisfaction

	Reported by:	
	fathers	mothers
Things worked out better than expected when (partner) became pregnant	59%	70%
Things going very well	29%	43%
Wants life to continue in much the same way	43%	49%*
Total sample (=100%)	362	365

*This difference did not reach the level of statistical significance.

Discussion

Eight times more fathers in our sample were teenagers than might have been expected from a sample of births to mothers of all ages, and more than three times as many were in the next youngest age group, 20 to 24 years (OPCS 1981a). In addition to being young, as we have seen, the members of our sample were mostly working-class, with relatively low earnings and quite high levels of unemployment. The majority who were married had married women already pregnant, so one might suppose there had been some pressure on them to get married quickly. Despite all these potentially adverse factors, the men expressed a high degree of satisfaction with marriage. Only 1% said they thought their marriage was unhappy, There are, of course, dangers in accepting people's statements on this subject at their face value. Nobody who has married only recently likes to admit that things are not going well or that they may have made a mistake. There is a natural tendency to gloss over any problems, so one has to look around for corroborative evidence of marital harmony. Nearly all the men said they helped their wives with at least some domestic tasks. Few seemed to regret their previous, more active, social life. Pursuing hobbies at home, helping around the house, and helping with the baby seemed in most cases to compensate amply for their previous freedom to drink with their friends in local pubs. In so far as they thought their wives had changed since becoming a mother, these changes were perceived as being mostly for the better. Achieving rapid maturity was highly regarded in a way it might not be in more middle-class circles, where preserving the freedom and anarchy of youth and adolescence for a longer period might be more highly valued.

In addition to being so pleased with marriage, they were also pleased with fatherhood, which again, with a young and not very well-off group of men might be thought surprising. Only 5% said they had been upset on originally learning of the pregnancy. Perhaps in the intervening year they had begun to forget how upset they really felt at the time, or perhaps they suppressed their feelings once the baby had actually arrived? Again, one looks for further evidence. Though most men approved of abortion in principle on very wide grounds, hardly any thought this was a relevant solution in their own case. Only a handful even suggested it to their partners as a possibility, and none had considered adoption. Nearly all claimed to help look after the baby at least occasionally, and nearly all said they felt personally responsible for the baby's welfare.

So, supposing that these young men are really as pleased with marriage and fatherhood as they claim to be, what might be the explanation for their perhaps unexpected degree of satisfaction?

One explanation might be family background. As we have seen, many of the men had parents who had married young and had a lot of children. So in getting married young themselves and having a child right away, they were behaving quite conventionally in relation to their own background. The fact that they did not intend to repeat this large family pattern lay in the future. Most of the men intended to have only two or three children themselves. Meanwhile, the marriage enabled them to get away from their crowded homes. Much of their social life, as we have seen, took place in pubs before, often less from choice than from a lack of space and privacy at home. Now two-thirds had a place of their own. This must surely have contributed a good deal to the satisfaction they voiced with their present way of life.

In addition to getting away from home, another more positive factor might have been at work. Can it be that the men in our sample have chosen marriage, fatherhood, and domestic life because they genuinely felt ready for it? Those who strongly did not, may have opted out of this situation at an earlier stage by recourse to birth control and abortion—a tribute to the improvement in the family planning and abortion services during the past decade. Hence the satisfaction expressed. This then is not the traditional captive audience of young men frogmarched into matrimony as a result of accidental pregnancy. Indeed, rather the other way round. Some, as we have seen, achieved marriage through pregnancy. If this is a realistic interpretation of these findings, then it suggests that there may at last be light at the end of the tunnel, and that we are well on the way to achieving the Mecca of the family planners, expressed in their slogan 'Every Child a Wanted Child' though that might be putting it a little strongly. Perhaps 'Every Child an Accepted or Tolerated Child' might be a more accurate if somewhat less exhilarating slogan.

Forty per cent of the men said they wanted a baby. In answer to another similar question, just over half of the men said they intended their partner to become pregnant then. One may conclude therefore that around half the men had a positive attitude to having a child at that time. At one level this is welcome news; but at the same time, their immaturity and their economic prospects both might suggest that it would have been wise to wait. This raises complex questions about the role of social policy in discouraging people from doing potentially damaging things they may feel impelled to do. In relation to smoking, drinking, and driving, many people would now accept that social policy does have a role to play, but with very young parenthood there is less consensus, and the issues seem less clear-cut to some people.

One-fifth of the men, as we have seen, were attempting to use birth control around the time their partner became pregnant. In addition to these men who were using a method, albeit inefficiently, there was another group of just over 10% of the sample who had used a method in the past but had had problems with it and had temporarily abandoned birth control or were between methods when the pregnancy occurred. These two groups must surely constitute the natural target for the next phase of family planning endeavour. Here is a group of young men whose motivation is established even though their practice is weak. What is the most effective way of bringing birth control services to young working-class men who are aware of their need for birth control without having any very clear idea of what to do about it? They are probably healthy enough at that age and do not see much of their GPs, most of whom anyway do not readily accept the role of distributors of male methods of contraception. Cossey (1979) notes that there is evidence from Holland, Sweden, and elsewhere, that brand advertising of male methods of contraception on television, commercial radio, in the cinema, and in the press may have an important role to play in contraceptive education. The Independent Broadcasting Authority's continued refusal to permit such advertising on television (while allowing advertising for beer despite anxieties about alcohol misuse in the community) is particularly damaging to the interests of this group and the health and welfare of their female partners.

The general picture that emerges from this survey is that these fathers indicate a high degree of satisfaction with their relationship with their partners, domestic life, and fatherhood. It may be that the delightful novelty of their situation was still uppermost in their minds at the time of interview. It may also be that this becomes modified in time in face of a more mobile and demanding child, further additions to the family and failure to improve standards of living in accordance with earlier ambitions and expectations. One can, however, conclude that in the initial phase at least, the attitudes of many of the current generation of young married men to family life are positive.

12 Discussion and conclusions. Some consequences for social policy.

A number of specific social policy consequences stem from some of these findings. The educational arrangements for the schoolgirl mothers varied widely (see Appendix 4). Some received home tuition for only one month, some for more than four months. Some had two hours teaching a week, some had as much as ten hours. Some had none at all. This may suggest the desirability of reviewing the present very arbitrary local authority educational arrangements for this group. The Joint Working Party on Pregnant Schoolgirls and Schoolgirl Mothers which reported in 1979 made similar observations and recommended that:

> 'Home tuition should be available without delay ... Where possible it should be based on home teaching centres.'

The inadequacy and ineffectiveness of current sex and birth control education given at schools is highlighted by this study. Among the schoolgirls in the study half had received some education of this kind. Despite this, nine of the ten became pregnant without deliberately intending to and only two of the ten were even attempting to use any form of birth control at the time they became pregnant. Among the 10% of the total sample who told us both that their pregnancy was unintended and that they were upset on first realising they were pregnant, again about half had received some birth control education at school, but only one quarter had attempted to use a method around the time they conceived, and this unsuccessfully. Once pregnant, three times as many of these women as in the rest of the sample considered having an abortion. It seems that the sex and birth control education at present available in some schools does not even prevent those becoming pregnant who are reluctant to embark on motherhood. An examination of the content of sex and birth control education currently available in schools is long overdue. This is particularly important given that the average age of first sexual experience of our sample was only 16.1 years. It may be, however, that the schools cannot expect to have much success in this field with a group of youngsters, many of whom are already deeply alienated from the school environment and nearly all of whom leave school at the first possible moment. It may be that the television and the media need to be more actively involved in this field if any progress is to be made and it is therefore particularly regrettable that the IBA has for so long been obstructive on this issue on the dubious grounds of not wishing to give offence to the public. This recommendation is also relevant to our findings about the young men in our sample. Half the men looked forward positively to having a baby when they did, but half were unenthusiastic and many of these had been making intermittent but not successful attempts

100

to use birth control. They were interested and motivated but ignorant and inexperienced. It seems extraordinary, given some of the feature films and other material that is deemed suitable for showing on the commercial channels, that birth control education and advertising should be virtually excluded. A change in the regulations permitting GPs to dispense condoms would also be helpful in providing an additional source of supply of contraceptives for young couples.

Some women within our sample, probably between 5% and 10%, would have preferred to have an abortion rather than become a mother so young. They were prevented from achieving their objective by their own inertia, the attitudes of family and friends, and the obstruction of some doctors who managed to prevent even some very young women who consulted them early in pregnancy from obtaining the abortions they requested. Probably between 3,000–6,000 unwanted births among teenage women could be prevented nationally if those doctors who objected to abortion in principle were obliged to make this important fact known to their patients (as recommended by witnesses to the Lane Committee on Abortion a decade ago) and if direct access abortion clinics were available.

The other side of this coin is that a few young women (see page 26) are nervous about coming early for ante-natal care in case pressure is brought to bear on them to have abortions they do not really wish to have. This underlines the importance of reassuring patients that their own views and opinions, whatever they may be, will be taken seriously within the limits permitted by the 1967 Abortion Act.

Most of the women who had considered adoption were satisfied with the decision they reached. Two women, however, whose babies were adopted later when they were older were not so satisfied, and some women who kept their babies then resented being trapped in poverty and unwanted domesticity. This suggests that there is still scope for realistic counselling, especially of young, poor, single women who may be contemplating adoption rather uncertainly. They need to think things out carefully well before the baby's birth so that adoption can take place immediately if it takes place at all, and they may need help in coming to terms with the very restricted lifestyle they may have to face if they decide to keep the baby after all.

Nearly all the young mothers had seen a GP and a health visitor. But few had seen a social worker. At the initial interview 6% of young mothers said they would have liked to discuss their problems with a social worker but had not had the opportunity to do so. They wanted to discuss housing, finance, marital problems and depression. Most of the women who had had this opportunity, said the social workers had proved helpful. It seems that there is a greater need for referral to social workers than GPs and health visitors are at present aware of, and they should be encouraged to consider such referrals when dealing with teenage mothers who appear to have social or marital problems. For example, nearly half of our teenage mothers who had separated from their husbands had experienced battering as had some who had not separated, and the majority had suffered episodes of depression or nerves. So this group would certainly benefit from such social worker contact even if only temporarily to help them over a bad patch.

Four-fifths of the young mothers declared themselves satisfied with the services they encountered at both their ante-natal and their baby clinics. But in each case around one-fifth had reservations. These two groups did not overlap although their complaints were similar—overcrowding, long waits, hurried attention which affected the quality of advice given them and their babies. In relation to ante-natal care, we concluded that there was a failure of management, and that patients not judged to be in a high risk category should be required to attend less frequently, but seen more promptly and offered more time, attention and discussion when they did come. In relation to the baby clinics, we concluded there might be room for improvement in the appointments systems but the real problem of too many clients and too few staff was unlikely to be solved without further resources being devoted to this service.

At both interviews, around a third of the teenage mothers regarded their current housing as unsuitable for their needs and about one in 20 reported that they moved frequently from one type of unsatisfactory accommodation to another. Much of this temporary accommodation was, if not council owned, then effectively council financed and some of it was in very poor condition. It is recommended that councils exercise much closer supervision over their emergency and 'short-term' housing to ensure that certain minimum standards of amenity are maintained.

The importance of housing provision as a stabilising factor in teenage marriage also emerged from this study, particularly in relation to the young fathers who on the whole were quite happy to lead a more restricted social life than before provided they had a home of their own in which to pursue their hobbies and domestic tasks. Previously, much of their social life had taken place in pubs and within their peer group, probably because pubs were the most accessible places to which to escape from overcrowded parental homes. Once they had independent homes of their own the attraction of the pub waned. One of the young separated mothers who had become reconciled with her husband, remarked on the improvement in their lives and her husband's temper as a result of being rehoused in a council flat. Improvements in housing and house furnishings played a large part in the hopes and expectations expressed by these young women when asked to reflect on the future.

Our investigation of the smoking habits of our sample showed that one-third of the young mothers who smoked wished to give up smoking, partly for health and partly for financial reasons. It is recommended that taxes on cigarettes be raised in order to reinforce this awareness and any additional revenue thus raised be spent on further publicising the health message since this may have already begun to make an impact on this age group.

The smoking study also illustrated the boredom and isolation that some of these mothers endured once they were trapped with young children away from family and friends. This suggests a need for a greater provision of day nurseries for young children and social clubs for young mothers, especially on or near housing estates. Young mothers' clubs might encourage teenage mothers to form self-help and baby sitting groups and thus give them a feeling of control over their own lives that so many lack at the moment. This lack of autonomy may also contribute to producing the depression and nerves reported by more than two-fifths of the women in our sample. They, however, ascribed these feelings to the responsibility of having a baby so young, to their sometimes dismal housing, poor relationships with their partners, loneliness, and poverty. In a fifth of the women who experienced depression or nerves, the condition was sufficiently severe to prevent them living normally and meeting other people. Not surprisingly, then a large number of young mothers also expressed the wish for part-time work. If this desire is to be satisfied, there needs to be a further expansion of part-time job opportunities for young unskilled or semi-skilled working-class women.

This conclusion leads to a consideration of the wider implications of the lack of any viable alternative to early motherhood for many of the young women in our sample. Even in present circumstances possibly a tenth of these women accepted the role of motherhood with marked reluctance. It is reasonable to suppose that this proportion would have been larger had attractive job opportunities been readily available to provide them with money and adult companionship. In so far as the prospects of work and money provide the motivation to postpone early motherhood, the current outlook is unpromising. For many young women early motherhood provides virtually the only opportunity to attain self-respect and adult status, even where this is undertaken in the most adverse circumstances. One young woman, separated from her hard drinking husband and now back with her baby in the overcrowded parental home, told us that her status within her family had improved since she had the baby, and, despite her domestic problems and debts, she was now happier than before she had the child.

A majority of teenagers are sexually experienced nowadays, but only a small minority (see, for example, Farrell, 1978; Dunnell, 1979) become teenage parents. Some assume this role in the absence of any more attractive alternatives and some others do so very reluctantly, having become pregnant by accident and having failed to obtain an abortion in time. These young women might have avoided becoming teenage mothers had we been able to offer them other sources of self-esteem, had we had a more effective system of contraceptive education, and birth control and abortion services more accessible to teenagers. Whether effective contraceptive education can be best accomplished through the schools, with the co-operation of the media, or with the help of specialist organisations like the Family Planning Association, the Brook Advisory Centres, Grapevine or similar, or a combination of all of these, remains to be determined, and constitutes a research area of importance. However, the expansion of existing birth control services specialising in advice for adolescents is obviously desirable and probably saves the community money even in the short run.

The majority of the teenagers in our sample, however, seemed pleased to become parents so soon and for this group social policy must aim at minimising the possible ill-effects of this for both parents and children. Better housing provision and a lessening of the young mothers' social isolation would do much to help. Money is another important issue. At the follow-up interview, more than half the mothers said that money was a problem for them, a quarter said they were in receipt of supplementary benefits, and nearly a quarter said they or their child went short of things they needed.

It would not be difficult to transform the situation of most of these young mothers if enough resources were devoted to this. The question to be determined is what priority they have in relation to other needy groups in the community. This is an issue of policy not research.

Appendix 1 The way the sample was selected

The sample was taken from births to teenage women that occurred during July 1979. This was done using a two-stage sample design.

The first stage was the selection of study areas. These were registration districts or groups of geographically contiguous registration districts in England and Wales. Registration districts were grouped so that there would be sufficient numbers of births to teenage women in an interviewer's area. Using data about the number of births to teenage women in each registration district during 1977, 117 primary sampling units (that is single or groups of registration districts) were created; in the smallest primary sampling unit there were 299 births to teenage women in 1977 and in the largest there were 1,596. The primary sampling units were divided into three size strata—those with a high, medium and low number of births to teenage women in 1977—and in each size strata, were listed on a north to south basis starting with those in Greater London and the metropolitan counties. The study areas were then selected from the three size strata with different sampling fractions (see Table A1).

The second stage was the selection of births to teenage women in each of the study areas. This was done using an appropriate sampling fraction, that is, one which meant that each birth had an equal chance of being selected taking both stages of the sample design into account.

Table A1 The sample design

	Stratum 1	Stratum 2	Stratum 3
Size (no. of births to teenage women in 1977)	299–375	376–700	701–1596
Sampling fraction (study areas)*	1/k	2/k	4/k
Sampling fraction (births to teenage women)	1	1/2	1/4
Quota sizes (no. of births to teenage women per month in 1977)	25–31	15–29	15–33
Stratum size (no. of primary sampling units)	38	70	9
Stratum mean	345.6	464.6	1082.7

* $k = 8.01$ and was calculated using the following equation:

$$\bar{x}_1 \times \frac{n_1}{k} + \bar{x}_2 \times \frac{n_2}{k/2} \times \tfrac{1}{2} + \bar{x}_3 \times \frac{n_3}{k/4} \times \tfrac{1}{4} = \text{set sample size}$$

where $\bar{x}$ = mean number of births per month to teenage women in primary sampling units in strata,

n = number of sampling units in strata,

and k = unknown constant.

Various combinations of size strata and sampling fractions were tried. The one which yielded the least variable quota sizes—this was considered important from a fieldwork point of view—was selected and is shown in Table A1.

The 26 study areas selected are shown in Table A2.

Table A2   The study areas

Area number	Registration district(s)
	Stratum 1
1	Gateshead/North Tyneside West
2	Hounslow/Richmond/Wandsworth
3	Melton Mowbray/Rutland/Corby/Kettering/Oundle and Thrapston/Stamford/Bourne/Grantham
4	Swansea
5	Surrey Mid-Eastern/Surrey Northern/Surrey South-Eastern/Surrey South-Western
	Stratum 2
6	Sunderland
7	Dewsbury/Huddersfield
8	Barnsley/Rotherham
9	Stockport/Trafford
10	Walsall/Sandwell
11	Islington/Haringey/Waltham Forest
12	Greenwich/Bexley
13	Carlisle/Wigton/Penrith/Appleby/Cockermouth/Whitehaven
14	Hull/Beverley/Pocklington/Bridlington
15	Boston/Caistor/East Elloe/Gainsborough/Horncastle/Lincoln/Louth/Sleaford/Spalding/Spilsby
16	Mansfield/Newark/Bosford/East Retford
17	Alcester/North Warwickshire/Nuneaton/Rugby/Shipston-on-Stour/Southam/Stratford/Warwick and Leamington
18	Ampthill/Bedford/Biggleswade/Leighton Buzzard/Aylesbury/North Buckinghamshire
19	Broxbourne/Dacorum/Elstree and Potters Bar/Hitchin/St. Albans/Watford/Stevenage
20	Neath/Ogwr
21	North-East Hampshire/Surrey North-Western
22	Southampton
	Stratum 3
23	Manchester
24	Birmingham
25	Central Cleveland
26	Leicestershire Central/Hinkley/Coalville/Loughborough/Market Harborough

To allow for the fact that the actual number of study areas varied from the expected number in each of the strata (see Table A3) the sampling fractions used to select births to teenage women were adjusted from those shown in Table A1. In study areas in stratum 1 one in every 19.22 births during the sampling period was removed from the sample; in study areas in strata 2 and 3 one in every 1.95 births and one in every 3.56 births, respectively, were included in the sample. Altogether 623 births to teenage women were selected.

Table A3   The expected and actual number of study areas

Stratum	Expected number*	Actual number
1	4.74	5
2	17.48	17
3	4.49	4

* The expected number of study areas was obtained by dividing the number of primary sampling units in a strata by the relevant sampling fraction, eg in strata 1 the expected number of study areas was 38/8.01.

Birth registration data about the age of the mother at the time of the baby's birth are regarded as confidential. To help preserve this confidentiality a condition of being able to draw our sample of births to teenage mothers was that it had to include a small number of ineligible births (that is, to women aged 20 and over). Forty-four births to older women were therefore included in the sample.

Appendix 2 The response of the mothers

The mothers of the sampled babies were sent a letter which gave them brief details of the survey and told them that an interviewer would be calling in the next few weeks. During September and October 1979, 533 (86%) of the 623 teenage mothers in the sample were successfully interviewed. The reason for failure are shown in Table A4.

Table A4   The response of the mothers

	Initial stage	Follow-up stage
	%	%
Successfully interviewed	86	89
Direct refusal	6	5
Inconvenient	2	1
Away all survey period	1	1
Out all calls	1	1
Moved/no trace	4	3
Number of women approached (= 100%)	623*	515

* The 44 women in the sample who were aged 20 and over were excluded from the analysis.

A third (35%) of the 533 teenage mothers were interviewed within ten weeks of their giving birth; two-fifths (38%) were interviewed in the tenth or eleventh week after they gave birth and just over a quarter (27%) were interviewed 12 or more weeks after they gave birth.

During these initial interviews the women were asked if they would be willing for an interviewer to call again in the future. The response was almost unanimously 'yes', only three respondents refusing the recall. Also excluded from the follow-up stage were the 15 women whose baby had died or been adopted before the initial interview. It was felt that a follow-up interview with this group might prove too distressing. Futhermore, many of the topics covered at this stage were not applicable to these women.

The 515 women who were eligible for the follow-up stage were sent a letter in June 1980 reminding them that an interviewer would be calling again and asking them to fill in a form giving their change of address, if any, and convenient times for an interviewer to call. During the following September and October 456 (89%) of them were successfully re-interviewed. Table A4 shows the reason why we failed to re-interview the remaining 11%.

Altogether 73% of the 623 teenage women in the sample were interviewed at both stages. This proportion rises to 77% if we exclude the women whose baby had died or been adopted before the initial interview.

How representative though are these women who responded to our survey? Comparison with OPCS data about births to women aged under 20 (OPCS 1981 and 1981b) did not reveal any bias in relation to their age or marital status. The proportion of their babies who died within a year of birth was, however, twice that expected from the national data (4% against 2%). Further comparisons, based on data collected from the birth registration forms of the sampled babies and during the initial stage of the study, also revealed a bias towards the native born, and the better off. This can be seen in Table A5.

Table A5   Some differences between responders and non-responders to the survey

	Responders	Non-responders
Initial stage		
Born in India, Pakistan, Bangladesh or Sri Lanka	4% (531)*	11% (90)
Partner born in West Indies	3% (531)	16% (56)
Baby adopted	† (533)	10% (91)
Follow-up stage‡		
Born in Great Britain	92% (455)	83% (151)
No educational qualifications	50% (456)	69% (62)
Last job before the 'survey' baby's birth classified as social class IV or V	44% (358)	59% (49)
Shares bathroom	3% (449)	11% (62)
Received help from partner with:		
washing up	57% (392)	42% (53)
household repairs	52% (392)	32% (53)
shopping	64% (392)	43% (53)
Received help in looking after the 'survey' baby from friends and neighbours	30% (453)	14% (59)

* The figures in brackets are the numbers on which the percentages are based.
† Less than 0.5%.
‡ The women whose baby had died or been adopted before the initial interview were omitted from the follow-up stage comparisons.

At both stages of the study structured questionnaires were used. Copies of these are available from the Institute for Social Studies in Medical Care, 14 South Hill Park, London NW3 2SB. The initial interviews took rather longer than the follow-up ones, on average 1.4 and 1.1 hours respectively. Most of the interviews 71% at the initial stage and 70% at the follow-up one, were carried out without other people present. An interpreter was used for 3% of the interviews at each stage.

Appendix 3 The response of the fathers

Where we had interviewed the mother of a 'survey' baby we wanted to interview the father. The mothers were therefore asked at the conclusion of their initial interview for the name and address of the 'survey' baby's father. Most of the women (84%) gave us this information; the proportion was 93% among those who were married when their 'survey' baby was registered but only 64% among those who were single at that time.

Altogether, we obtained the names and addresses of 446 men. Of these, 83% were successfully interviewed between October 1979 and January 1980. The reasons for failure are shown in Table A6. So, of the 623 men who were eligible for inclusion in the study, 59% were ultimately interviewed—at the initial stage.

Table A6   The response of the men

	%
Successfully interviewed	83
Direct refusal	7
Inconvenient	2
Away all survey period	2
Out all calls	4
Moved, no trace	2
Ineligible (informant denied paternity)	*
Number of men (= 100%)	446

*Less than 0.5%.

As with the women, a structured questionnaire was used. Copies of this questionnaire are also available from the Institute for Social Studies in Medical Care, 14 South Hill Park, Hampstead, London NW3 2SB. The interviews took 1.1 hours on average and most (75%) of them were carried out without other people present. An interpreter was used for 1% of the interviews.

The representatives of the fathers' sample

The response rate obtained with the fathers' sample was comparatively low. Can we identify any specific biases?

Comparison with OPCS data (OPCS, 1981b), about births to women aged under 20 showed that men who were single when their 'survey' baby was born are under-represented in the sample; the proportion was 23% which is only just over half that expected from national data. Other comparisons, based on data collected from the birth certificates of the 'survey' babies and during the initial interviews with the women showed that men aged under 19 or over 23, men in unskilled jobs, and men born

110

in the West Indies are also under-represented in the sample. Furthermore, there was some indication that the men we failed to interview were less pleased about becoming a father and were less involved in baby care than the men we managed to interview (see Table A7). It is likely, therefore, that the data obtained during the interviews with the fathers give a more favourable view of young fatherhood than is really justified.

Table A7 Some differences between fathers who responded and those who did not

	Data from mothers' questionnaire			
	Responders		Non-responders	
The men's characteristics:				
aged under 19	9%	(367)	18%	(158)
aged 24 and over	20%	(367)	30%	(158)
classified as social class V	9%	(348)	20%	(184)*
born in the West Indies	1%	(369)	7%	(217)*
Mother's view of her partner's attitude to the pregnancy:				
mixed or upset feelings	24%	(368)	39%	(150)
Mother's report of her partner's involvement in baby care. Partner:				
never changed the baby's nappy	26%	(355)	45%	(119)
never fed the baby	5%	(338)	18%	(109)
never bathed the baby	64%	(355)	79%	(119)
never dressed the baby	30%	(355)	41%	(119)
never looked after the baby while she had been out for an hour or more	22%	(355)	44%	(119)
never taken the baby out alone	49%	(355)	61%	(119)
Proportion of single fathers who:				
have never seen the baby	1%	(75)	36%	(99)
have seen the baby but not in the last 7 days	8%	(75)	20%	(99)
gave no financial help	21%	(73)	60%	(99)

Figures in brackets are the numbers on which the percentages are based.
*Includes data from birth certificates for non-responders at the mother's stage.

111

Appendix 4 The schoolgirls and their boyfriends

Within the general category of teenagers, the schoolgirls are a distinct group due to their legal and educational status. They are obliged to receive some form of education whether they like it or not, unlike their older sisters. Moreover, as a result of (at time of writing) two conflicting legal judgements which have to be resolved by a final judgement in the House of Lords, there is intense public and professional controversy (see, for example, British Medical Journal, 1985 and 1985a; and Lancet, 1985) about whether girls aged under 16 should be permitted to receive birth control advice and instruction without the express consent of their parents. This controversy is unlikely to be ended by the decision of the law lords, whichever way the judgement goes, because it is based on irreconcilable views about the importance or otherwise of medical confidentiality, and how far children may reasonably be held to be the property of their parents. Thus, despite the fact that our numbers are small and preclude any comparisons being made between them and the rest of the sample, we thought it worth including a descriptive account of a group that is much in the public eye.

The first interview

The families of origin

In our sample of 533 teenage mothers, there were ten schoolgirl mothers. Two were aged 14 years at the time of their baby's birth and the remainder were aged 15 years. They came from unusually large families. The average family size was five, with one girl having seven and another 12 siblings. Already the ten girls had 27 nephews and nieces between them. One girl's mother became pregnant again soon after she did and another girl had two siblings who had both given birth to their first child at 15 years. On average the girls themselves eventually wanted three or four children each.

How far is this picture part of a large family sub-culture rather than a sign of social deviance? The schoolgirls' mothers also started having children very young. Two were teenagers at the time, and five were in their early twenties, as were three of the fathers. So it could be argued that these girls were simply repeating a family pattern. Against this interpretation, one must set the fact that none of their mothers was pleased to learn of the pregnancy, and half of them were positively shocked and upset on hearing the news:

'She went mad—she said I'd ruined my life—but she's glad now.'

'She was heartbroken.'

'She was hurt, couldn't believe it could happen to me, upset that her daughter was pregnant at 14.'

One mother, however, was quite philosophical about the event:

'She said it was one of those things and she was very helpful.'

Generally the reaction of the fathers was similar to that of the mothers, with the exception of one West Indian father who was positively pleased about his daughter's pregnancy. On the whole, however, the parents evidently hoped for something different for their daughters.

All the parents were born in England and Wales except for two sets who were born in the West Indies. One father had died, one was unemployed and five worked in a variety of unskilled or semi-skilled jobs. Of the remainder, one was a manager, one a publican and one a farmer. All but two of the parents, one of whom was widowed, were still together. All the girls said that they got on well with their mothers and only two said that they did not get on well with their fathers.

All but one of the parents gave their daughters financial support, mostly on a regular basis. Nearly all the girls were dependent on heavy subsidies from their parents for housing, maintainence, baby care and baby sitting. The girls' awareness of the social costs to the family of their having a baby so young seemed to be almost non-existent. One remarked:

'It's all worked out fine with my mum looking after her, and I have the best of both worlds. I love having her and just carrying on as usual at school.'

School

School evoked little enthusiasm, although half of the sample hoped to take some public examinations in the future. The amount of compensatory education they received whilst pregnant varied widely, as did their opinion of it.

Six girls had returned to school full-time, and two more said that they were about to go back. But two said they felt it was more important to be at home with the baby, although they saw a home tutor occasionally. In all, seven girls had had some individual tuition during pregnancy. The number of hours per week varied from two to ten, averaging about six hours per week. The number of weeks for which this lasted also varied widely, generally from four to 18 weeks—though in one case tuition was supplied for 30 weeks. Again, opinions about the tuition differed greatly. Three girls were enthusiastic about it. For example:

'The teacher was very helpful and I found the work interesting. If I had any (personal) problems I could talk to her.'

Others were indifferent or positively disliked it:

'They were a waste of time. She (the tutor) used to sit and watch TV all the time.'

Asked what they wanted to do when they left school, half of the girls did not know at all, and others mentioned typing, machining, and nursery nursing. Two girls had previously intended to nurse. They realised that, with a baby, this was no longer possible, but could think of nothing else. However, one girl, encouraged by her school, hope to train as a silversmith.

Birth control

Research brought its usual puzzles. Half of the girls had had sex education at school, and four out of the ten had also discussed birth control. Only one girl actually intended to become pregnant. Despite this, only two were using any form of birth control when they became pregnant. When asked why they had not used birth control, some gave more than one reason. Two said that they 'didn't know' why they had not, three said that they didn't think about birth control at all or that 'you think it will never happen to you'. Two said that they did not realise it was possible to get pregnant so quickly, since 'it was only once' or 'I'd only been with him three times'. One girl said she simply 'didn't know any methods', so took a chance. Another did likewise because they 'didn't enjoy it so much using a condom or whatever you call it'.

However, only three girls said that they were upset when they first thought they might be pregnant. Three more had mixed feelings, worrying chiefly about being under age or about their parents' reactions. One said that she had no reaction 'apart from thinking I could have it adopted if I was (pregnant)' while the remainder said they were pleased.

The two girls who had used birth control at the time they became pregnant had both had sex education and birth control instruction at school. One had relied on the sheath and withdrawal, but not regularly. The other had relied on the sheath alone but now thought the method unreliable.

Eight girls said that they now knew enough about birth control, having discussed the matter with their GP, hospital doctor, midwife, health visitor or social worker since becoming pregnant. All but two girls thought that both men and women ought to be responsible for taking precautions to avoid pregnancy, rather than just one or other of them. 'It saves anything from going wrong' said one girl, presumably not referring to her own case, 'if one fails, the other is bound to work'.

An air of fatalism seems to pervade the whole subject of birth control. Whether intended or not, pregnancy in these cases just seemed to happen, and the girls went ahead with it, possibly because none of the educational or work alternatives seemed to be very attractive. Having a baby, even so young, constituted an acceptable lifestyle in their circle, and one that conferred more status and perhaps more genuine satisfaction than did anything else open to them.

The partners

The mothers were asked about the fathers of their babies. They were also young. Two fathers, being 15 and 16 years of age, were still at school at the time of the interview with the mother. Two others were aged 18, three were 17 and three were 19 years of age. These men had all left school at the earliest possible moment. In fact, one was described by his partner as being 'kicked out at 14 years'. Of another it was said:

'He never went to school hardly—he just didn't used to go.'

All the men were born in England and Wales except for one born in Eire and one in the West Indies. Most of these young fathers were in unskilled or semi-skilled jobs. One was unemployed.

Five of the young fathers were described as being pleased on being told of the pregnancy, while three had mixed feelings and two were upset. All but these last two had discussed marriage with the girl and had expressed the intention of marrying her when she was older. Seven girls thought that they and the father would get married in due course and one was uncertain.

The young fathers' degree of participation in baby care and domestic tasks seemed surprisingly high given that opportunities for this were limited, since most of the fathers still lived away from the mother with their own parents. Four were described as looking after the baby in a variety of ways frequently, and others did so occasionally. Three fathers also helped with the shopping, cooking, washing-up and washing.

Seven fathers contributed financially, three of these on a regular basis, the sums mentioned being five pounds per week, seven pounds per week and £15 per week. One contributed by buying whatever the baby needed. One said that he would contribute if he earned any money. One girl said 'I'm not bothered because I'm not going out with him for his money', but another said she was afraid 'he would have a legal right to her (the baby) if he helped me financially and I don't want that.' Asked how, if at all, their relationship with the baby's father had changed since becoming pregnant, three girls said that there had been no change, and five said that they had become closer. But two said their relationship had deteriorated.

Motherhood

Although half the girls said they had suffered from depression or nerves since returning home with the baby, most thought that the coming of the baby had improved the quality of their lives, giving them 'something to do' as one girl remarked, or giving them something of their own as several others remarked. Perhaps this reflects a large family lifestyle, where everything is communal and few things can be said to belong specifically to any one member of the family, at least when they are all young. Clothes, toys, books and sports equipment all get passed down the line, and feelings of personal possession are dissipated. But the baby indisputably belongs to one person and is her possession.

There was no sense of regret about the passing of youth. Great store seemed to be set by maturing quickly. 'I used to be a tomboy/go to discos/go round with my mates'—but not any more. To have rapidly outgrown that childish stage and to have entered into these new family responsibilities as early as possible seemed to be looked upon favourably.

The girls also appeared cheerful about their prospects. They did not think that they would have any great problems in the near future. They thought that things had worked out well, and did not believe that either they or their parents had, or would, suffer as a result of having their babies at 14 or 15 years of age.

The question that immediately suggests itself is how far this seeming complacency is merely a reflection of the novelty of their situation. Did this euphoria wear off later when the children were older and beginning to be mobile?

One year later

Two of the mothers were now married, two were cohabiting and the remainder were single. One of the single girls was still under age but expecting to marry when she was 16. Four girls had broken up with their boyfriends, sometimes with bitterness:

'I just don't want to have anything to do with him any more. I just don't want to.'

One girl explained that she had not tried to obtain any money from the father because:

'I think it would give him more of a hold on her and I don't want him to be able to say, "I did this and that for her". I wouldn't want him ever to be able to take her away.'

Another young father had acquired a new girlfriend, on whom he now spent his money:

'I've tried (to get money from him) but he just says he's not going to give it to me.'

Sadly, one baby died during the year. This was described as a 'cot death' and had taken place at a childminder's house, where the childminder looked after two other babies as well. This young mother, however, seemed to have made a good recovery from the tragedy. She described her own health as fairly good and said she had not suffered from depression or nerves as a result of this experience, though she had reported doing so at the time of our first visit, when the baby was still alive and apparently doing well and gaining weight rapidly.

This young mother had returned to her old school briefly, left without passing any examinations and obtained a factory job at £33 per week. She had recently married the father of the baby and they had moved into a council flat. With two incomes coming in and no baby to support, she said she felt better off than ever before and seemed quite pleased with life. She expressed the view that it would have been more difficult to be rehoused had the baby lived:

'We couldn't have had the flat with her. We would have had a long wait for a house.'

She told the interviewer that she and her husband were now saving up to buy carpets and hoped to have another baby after an interval of two or three years. They intended to have four children eventually, but meanwhile she was on the pill and now felt she knew enough about birth control, having asked her GP for advice on the subject.

This was a young woman who started having sex at the age of 14 years, had not intended to have a baby when she did, was upset when she found she was pregnant and had considered abortion. She had, however, been dissuaded from this by her boyfriend and mother. Now, married, rehoused, working and independent, she felt cheerful:

'We're on our way now. We haven't everyone else on to us all the time, so we get on much better.'

Another young mother seemed less happy and declined to be interviewed a second time. The interviewer observed:

'I understand that they have had little or no help or money from the DHSS and I felt that this had influenced their decision on refusing the interview.'

This was a mother who had had her first baby at 15 years. Due to the irregularity of her periods, she had not thought to visit her doctor until she was seven months pregnant. She had considered having the baby adopted, but when it was born, decided against this. She and the baby's 16 year old father were expecting to marry as soon as she had reached her 16th birthday.

At the time of the first interview, she had described her way of life very positively and said she hoped it would continue in much the same way. She had discussed birth control problems with the hospital social worker and visited a family planning clinic. She felt she knew enough about the subject and had told our interviewer that she did not intend to have another baby for five years, though she hoped to have four children eventually.

However, things had not gone according to plan. Since the last interview, she had had a second baby and had not, after all, married the boyfriend. She and the children lived in her parents' council house, along with three of her seven siblings and a nephew.

Family planning

Two other young mothers were pregnant again at the time of the second interview. Both said this pregnancy had been intended. One mother was now married: the other was pregnant by a new boyfriend, but the previous boyfriend still visited his baby at her home almost daily.

Five of the young women were using contraception—two had had IUDs fitted and the others relied on the pill, the sheath and the cap. Two said they were not using any contraceptive methods as they had no steady boyfriends. One added:

'My mother doesn't believe in it, in any form of birth control.'

All except two of the women said they thought they now knew enough about birth control. Of the two who did not, one was pregnant again and said she wanted to know more about the side effects of the pill. The other young woman had changed from the pill to the cap because she believed the pill had started off her depression. She now wanted to find out 'whether there was anything better'.

Depression

All the nine young mothers we were able to interview said their physical health had been quite good during the past year, but five said they had suffered episodes of depression or nerves. One said she thought it was due to a deteriorating relationship with the baby's father. She objected to his habit of going out without her on Friday nights and they had quarrelled continuously. She wondered whether he would abandon her and the baby and this had depressed her. Another girl, who was now pregnant again, ascribed the depression to extreme boredom. This had also led her to take up smoking:

117

'When I haven't got any fags, I get depressed, really fed up.'

Another young mother became depressed when she compared her situation with those of her contemporaries who were able to work, earn money and buy their own clothes. They were also able to enjoy some social life and were not tied to the home. Some of this feeling was echoed by another young mother, who said:

'It's the responsibility of having a baby at this age. You can't think about yourself any more, you've got to consider the baby's welfare as well.' It affects me, being on my own.'

Only one of the five had consulted her GP about her condition. He had talked to her about her problems and advised her to rest more. She said this discussion had been helpful and she was now feeling much better. The others felt that they themselves had to solve the problems that lay at the root of their depression, or that doctors could not help with problems of this kind:

'I don't think I can really talk to him. I keep thinking I'll get over it ...'

'I didn't think of telling anyone. I don't think it's really got a lot to do with the doctor.'

These two were still suffering from depression or nerves at the time of the second interview, but were hoping things would improve eventually.

Housing

Five young mothers—two married, two single and one cohabiting—had been rehoused by the local council. Several of these had moved many times in the course of the year. One had started off in a 'mother and baby' home and had moved back to her parents, before being rehoused by the council. Another had left her parent's home after several rows and moved in with her boyfriend's parents: from there into council 'half-way' accommodation and finally into their own council flat. Some had been rehoused from parents' overcrowded homes or from other kinds of unsuitable accommodation. Most of the others were still with their parents and siblings, with their names down on council waiting lists.

Education and jobs

Three girls were still at school at the time of the second interview. One was intending to take 'A' levels and become a computer operator. Another said she had only returned temporarily as she was getting married in three months' time. The third girl's comment was:

'I can't wait to leave.'

One girl had taken some CSE exams and was now pursuing a pre-nursing course at a further education college. Others were working part-time, or were looking for jobs. Only three girls said they were experiencing, or had experienced money problems—a reflection, perhaps of the generous subsidies received from their parents.

Overall impressions

None of the mothers interviewed thought things had gone worse than expected since the time they first found out they were pregnant. Seven actually said things had gone better than anticipated. Two of these mentioned being rehoused as the main reason for their sense of well-being. Other reasons included receiving more help from their parents than they had expected, the baby's father 'sticking by them' and the decision of the grandparents in one case to adopt their grandchild, leaving the young mother free to pursue her own life once again.

Six of the young mothers said they were pleased they had the baby when they did, despite their extreme youth. Two had reservations:

'It's worked out really well, but I wish I'd had her when I was older . . .'

'I was too young. I think I should have done something, worked, saved money and got everything before I had a baby.'

Discussion

At the conclusion of the first set of interviews, when the babies were about four months old, we noted how cheerful the young mothers seemed about their future prospects. They thought the babies had improved the quality of their lives and could foresee no great problems in the near future. We wondered how far this seeming complacency was a reflection of the novelty of their situation.

By the second interview, one year or more later, several of these young women had had severely adverse experiences. Nonetheless, most were still satisfied with their lives and their choices. It is pleasing that these young mothers are still so satisfied, but it has to be said that their prospects do not seem very promising to an outsider. This raises all kinds of questions about how far it is ever possible to make judgements about the quality of peoples' lives. It also raises questions about the quality of the responses. After the experiences some of these girls have had, can they really believe they did the right thing in having a baby at 14 or 15 years, or is it simply necessary for them to say this in order to avoid feelings of dejection and failure? Expectations are another aspect of this, if life does not seem to offer a great deal in other respects, then perhaps having a baby, even so young, has its compensations?

Social policy conclusions are not easy to arrive at in this context. Despite the availability of birth control advice and help, three of these ten very young girls became pregnant again almost immediately. In two cases, this second pregnancy was stated to be intended. Where motivation is absent, it is doubtful whether improving the quality and scope of birth control services will have more than a marginal effect.

The general conclusion after two interviews seems to be that it is difficult to change attitudes to having babies so young, if this be thought desirable, without also changing much else about these women's lives—in particular, their hopes of a worthwhile and enjoyable alternative way of life. At the present time such prospects for young women with little education and few skills seem to be remote.

References

ALAN GUTTMACHER INSTITUTE (1976) *Eleven million teenagers; what can be done about the epidemic of adolescent pregnancies in the United States* New York: Alan Guttmacher Institute.

BALDWIN J A and OLIVER J E (1975) 'Epidemiological and family characteristics of severely abused children' *British Journal of Preventive and Social Medicine 4* 205–221.

BOLTON F C (1980) *The pregnant adolescent* Beverley Hills: Sage Publications.

BRITISH MEDICAL JOURNAL (1975) 'Pregnancy in adolescence' *British Medical Journal 3* 665–666.

BRITISH MEDICAL JOURNAL (1985) 'Teenage confidence and consent' *British Medical Journal 290* 144–145.

BRITISH MEDICAL JOURNAL (1985a) 'GMC amends advice on contraception and under 16s' *British Medical Journal 290* 653.

BROOK EDUCATION AND PUBLICATIONS UNIT (1981) *The consequences of teenage sexual activity* London: Brook Advisory Centres.

BROWN, G W and HARRIS, T (1978) *Social origins of depression* London: Tavistock Publications.

BURY, J (1984) *Teenage pregnancy in Britain* London: Birth Control Trust.

CARTWRIGHT, A (1976) *How many children?* London: Routledge and Kegan Paul.

CARTWRIGHT, A (1978) *Recent trends in family building and contraception* London: HMSO.

CARTWRIGHT, A (1979) *The dignity of labour?* London: Tavistock Publications.

CARTWRIGHT, A and ANDERSON, R (1981) *General practice revisited* London: Tavistock Publications.

CHAMBERLAIN, R, CHAMBERLAIN G, HOWLETT, B and CLAIREAUX A (1975) *British Births Survey 1970 Vol. 1* London: Heineman Medical Books.

CLARKE, J, MACPHERSON, B V and HOLMES, D R (1982) 'Cigarette smoking and external locus of control among young adolescents' *Journal of health and social behaviour 23* 253–259.

CLARKE, M and WILLIAMS, A J (1979) 'Depression in women after perinatal death' *Lancet i* 916–917.

COSSEY, D (1979) *Teenage birth control. The case for the condom* London: Brook Advisory Centres.

CENTRAL STATISTICAL OFFICE (1980) *Social trends 11* London: HMSO.

CENTRAL STATISTICAL OFFICE (1982) *Social trends 13* London: HMSO.

COMMITTEE ON ONE PARENT FAMILIES (1974) *Report* London: HMSO.

DUNNELL, K (1979) *Family Formation 1976* London: HMSO.

ELSTER, A B and PANZARINE, S (1981) 'The adolescent father' *Seminars in Perinatology 5* 39–51.

EUROPEAN COLLABORATIVE COMMITTEE FOR CHILD HEALTH (1983) *Teenage mothers* Liverpool: The Childrens Research Fund.

FARRELL, C (1978) *My mother said* ... London: Routledge and Kegan Paul.

FURSTENBURG, F F (1976) *Unplanned parenthood. The social consequences of teenage childbearing* New York: The Free Press.

GINSBERG, S and BROWN, G W (1981) 'No time for depression' in Mechanic, D (eds) *Psycho-social epidemiology: symptoms, illness behaviour and health seeking* New York: Neal Watson Academic Publishers.

HALL, M H, CHING, P, and MACGILLIVRAY, I (1980) 'Is routine antenatal care worthwhile?' *Lancet 2* 78–80.

HOLLINGSWORTH, D R and KREUTNER, A K K (1980) 'Teenage pregnancy. Solutions are evolving' *The New English Journal of Medicine 303* 516–518.

JOINT WORKING PARTY ON PREGNANT SCHOOLGIRLS AND SCHOOL-GIRL MOTHERS (1979) *Pregnant at school* London: National Council for One Parent Families.

KIERNAN, K E (1980) 'Teenage motherhood—associated factors and consequences—the experiences of a British birth cohort' *Journal of Biosocial Science 12* 393–405.

KLERMAN, L S (1980) 'Adolescent pregnancy: a new look at a continuing problem' *American Journal of Public Health 70* 776–778.

LANCET (1985) 'Contraception and the under-16s' *Lancet i* 827.

LAW COMMISSION (1981) *The financial consequences of divorce* London: HMSO.

MACFARLANE, A and MUGFORD, M (1984) *Birth counts: statistics of pregnancy and childbirth Vol. 1* London: HMSO.

MORRELL, D C, AVERY, A J and WATKINS, C J (1980) 'Management of minor illness' *British Medical Journal 280* 769–771.

O'BRIEN, M and SMITH, C (1981) 'Womens views and experiences of ante-natal care' *The Practitioner 225* 123–125.

OFFICE OF POPULATION CENSUSES AND SURVEYS (1977) *Population trends 10* London: HMSO.

OFFICE OF POPULATION CENSUSES AND SURVEYS (1981) 'Infant and perinatal morality' *OPCS Monitor DH3 81/1.*

OFFICE OF POPULATION CENSUSES AND SURVEYS (1981a) *Birth statistics 1979* London: HMSO.

OFFICE OF POPULATION CENSUSES AND SURVEYS (1981b) *General household survey 1979* London: HMSO.

OFFICE OF POPULATION CENSUSES AND SURVEYS (1981c) *Abortion Statistics 1979* London: HMSO.

OFFICE OF POPULATION CENSUSES AND SURVEYS (1981d) 'Cigarette smoking 1972–1980' *OPCS Monitor GHS 81/2.*

OFFICE OF POPULATION CENSUSES AND SURVEYS (1982) *Population trends 28* London: HMSO.

OFFICE OF POPULATION CENSUSES AND SURVEYS (1982a) Infant and perinatal mortality *OPCS Monitor DH3 82/3.*

OFFICE OF POPULATION CENSUSES AND SURVEYS (1982b) *Birth statistics 1980* London: HMSO.

OFFICE OF POPULATION CENSUSES AND SURVEYS (1982c) *General household survey 1980* London: HMSO.

OFFICE OF POPULATION CENSUSES AND SURVEYS (1984) 'Live births during 1983 by mothers age, legitimacy and birth order' *OPCS Monitor FM1 84/4.*

OFFICE OF POPULATION CENSUSES AND SURVEYS (1984a) *General household survey 1982* London: HMSO.

OSBOURNE, G K, HOWART, R C L and JORDAN, M M (1981) 'The obstetric outcome of teenage pregnancy' *British Journal of Obstetrics and Gynaecology 88* 215–221.

PARKE, R D, POWER, T G and FISHER, J (1980) 'The adolescent fathers impact on the mother' *Journal of Social Issues 36* 88–106.

REID, D (1982) 'School sex education and the causes of unintended teenage pregnancies—a review' *Health Education Journal 41* 4–11.

RICHARDS, M P H (1981) 'Post-divorce arrangements for children, a pyschological perspective' *Journal of Social Welfare Law* 133–151.

RIMMER, L (1981) *Families in focus: marriage, divorce and family patterns* London: Study Commission on the Family.

ROTHENBERG, P B and VARGO, P E (1981) 'Relationship between age of mother and child health and development' *American Journal of Public Health 71* 810–817.

RUSSELL, J K (1981) 'No Joy in the Youth Club' *The Guardian* September 1st.

RUSSELL, J K (1982) *Early teenage pregnancy* Edinburgh: Churchill Livingstone.

RUTTER, M (1979) *Changing youth in a changing society* London: Nuffield Provincial Hospital Trust.

SMITH, S M, HANSON R and NOBLE, S (1973) 'Parents of battered babies: a controlled study' *British Medical Journal 4* 388–391.

TAYLOR, B, WADSWORTH, J and BUTLER, N (1983) 'Teenage mothering: hospitalizations and accidents during the first five years' *Archives of Disease in Childhood 58* 6–11.

WILSON, F (1980) 'Antecedents of adolescent pregnancy' *Journal of Biosocial Science 12* 141–152.

WOLKIND, S N and KRUK, S (1985) Teenage pregnancy and motherhood *Journal of the Royal Society of Medicine 78* 112–5.

ZACKLER, J and BRADSTREET, W (1975) *The teenage pregnant girl* Illinois: Charles Thomas.

Printed in the UK for HMSO by Hobbs the Printers of Southampton
(3501) Dd738529 C10 2/86 G381